'Weaving together original contributions from law, ethics, theology and economics, this book provides many fresh insights into the vexed questions surrounding markets and healthcare – an integrative tour de force!'

Professor Bill Fulford, *University of Oxford, UK*

'Healthcare marketisation generates superheated controversy. But here is the cool consideration and balanced debate that is needed as a response. This collection is multifaceted, analytically rich and packed with insights.'

Professor Alan Cribb, *King's College London, UK*

'Markets make good servants but bad masters. But what forms of service can they perform and what evils of mastery do they threaten? These wide-ranging essays address those questions in politically and theologically challenging ways.'

Professor Albert Weale, *UCL, UK*

'A significant contribution to bioethics. The topic is timely, the writing brief and clear, and the ideas insightful. It is very balanced, incorporating many perspectives (from Hayek to Marx), and many disciplines (including medicine, economics, philosophy, and theology). I highly recommend it.'

Professor Daniel Sulmasy, *Georgetown University, USA*

Marketisation, Ethics and Healthcare

How does the market affect and redefine healthcare? The marketisation of Western healthcare systems has now proceeded well into its fourth decade. But the nature and meaning of the phenomenon has become increasingly opaque amidst changing discourses, policies and institutional structures. Moreover, ethics has become focussed on dealing with individual, clinical decisions and neglectful of the political economy which shapes healthcare.

This interdisciplinary volume approaches marketisation by exploring the debates underlying the contemporary situation and by introducing reconstructive and reparative discourses. The first part explores contrary interpretations of 'marketisation' on a systemic level, with a view to organisational-ethical formation and the role of healthcare ethics. The second part presents the marketisation of healthcare at the level of policy-making, discusses the ethical ramifications of specific marketisation measures and considers the possibility of reconciling market forces with a covenantal understanding of healthcare. The final part examines healthcare workers' and ethicists' personal moral standing in a marketised healthcare system, with a view to preserving and enriching virtue, empathy and compassion.

Fostering rich reflection on the moral implications of a marketised healthcare system, this book is suitable for health professionals and for academics and students interested in the health sciences, medical ethics and law, social and public policy, philosophy and theology.

Therese Feiler is the postdoctoral researcher with the Oxford Healthcare Values Partnership in the Faculty of Theology and Religion and Research Fellow at Harris Manchester College, University of Oxford, UK.

Joshua Hordern leads the Oxford Healthcare Values Partnership and is Associate Professor of Christian Ethics in the Faculty of Theology and Religion and a Fellow of Harris Manchester College, University of Oxford, UK.

Andrew Papanikitas is NIHR Academic Clinical Lecturer in General Practice in the Department of Primary Care Health Sciences and Research Fellow at Harris Manchester College, University of Oxford, UK.

Routledge Key Themes in Health and Society

www.routledge.com/Routledge-Key-Themes-in-Health-and-Society/book-series/RKTHS

Available titles include

The Story of Nursing in British Mental Hospitals
Echoes from the corridors
Niall McCrae and Peter Nolan

Living with Mental Disorder
Insights from qualitative research
Jacqueline Corcoran

A New Ethic of 'Older'
Subjectivity, Surgery and Self-stylization
Bridget Garnham

Social Theory and Nursing
Edited by Martin Lipscomb

Older Citizens and End-of-Life Care
Social work practice strategies for adults in later life
Malcolm Payne

Digital Technologies and Generational Identity
ICT Usage Across the Life Course
Sakari Taipale, Terhi-Anna Wilksa and Chris Gilleard

Partiality and Justice in Nursing Care
Marita Nordhaug

Forthcoming titles include

Negotiating Ageing
Critical Narratives for Cultural Adaptation
Simon Biggs

Marketisation, Ethics and Healthcare

Policy, Practice and Moral Formation

Edited by Therese Feiler,
Joshua Hordern and
Andrew Papanikitas

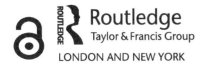

Routledge
Taylor & Francis Group

LONDON AND NEW YORK

First published 2018
by Routledge
4 Park Square, Milton Park, Abingdon, Oxon OX14 4RN
605 Third Avenue, New York, NY 10017

First issued in paperback 2023

Routledge is an imprint of the Taylor & Francis Group, an informa business

British Library Cataloguing-in-Publication Data
A catalogue record for this book is available from the British Library

Library of Congress Cataloging-in-Publication Data
A catalog record for this book has been requested

ISBN: 978-1-03-256999-4 (pbk)
ISBN: 978-1-138-73573-6 (hbk)
ISBN: 978-1-315-18635-1 (ebk)

DOI: 10.4324/9781315186351

Typeset in Times New Roman
by Apex CoVantage, LLC

οὐδεὶς δύναται δυσὶ κυρίοις δουλεύειν
Matthew 6:24

Contents

Acknowledgements

This book represents a collaboration which is international, national, and local. We have enjoyed close partnership with colleagues from Australia to Bahrain, from across the UK, and from various departments of the University of Oxford, namely the Faculty of Theology and Religion, the Nuffield Department of Primary Care Health Sciences, the Faculty of Law, the Blavatnik School of Government, and Ethox in the Nuffield Department of Population Health.

As editors, we gladly acknowledge funding from the British Academy to support this partnership in the form of a British Academy Rising Star Engagement Award (EN150004). This award was made to Joshua Hordern to enable academic and knowledge exchange collaboration with the Royal Society of Medicine Open and Primary Care Sections, represented by Andrew Papanikitas, formerly President of the Open Section. We are particularly grateful to Prof. Vivian Nutton, this project's British Academy champion, who provided wise guidance and participated in the project at various stages. We also are delighted to acknowledge support for Joshua Hordern and Therese Feiler from the Wellcome Trust Institutional Strategic Support Fund at the University of Oxford (105605/Z/14/Z) and the Arts and Humanities Research Council (AH/N009770/1).

To these funding bodies and colleagues, near and far, and to the editorial team at Routledge, especially Carolina Antunes, we hereby express our heartfelt thanks.

Finally, we are grateful for the continuing support of The Oxford Research Centre in the Humanities and for the community of Harris Manchester College, which has provided such an excellent home for this interdisciplinary research and engagement.

T.F., J.H., A.P.
August 2017
Harris Manchester College
University of Oxford Healthcare Values Partnership
www.healthcarevalues.ox.ac.uk

Contributors

Miran Epstein received his MD in 1987 from the Sackler School of Medicine, Tel Aviv University. He later completed his PhD at the Cohn Institute for the History and Philosophy of Science and Ideas, Tel Aviv University, having written his thesis on the history of contemporary medical ethics. Miran Epstein has published extensively on a wide spectrum of topics in medical ethics and is currently writing a book expounding on the argument he makes in this volume. At present, he is Reader in Medical Ethics at Barts and The London School of Medicine and Dentistry, Queen Mary University of London.

Therese Feiler is the postdoctoral researcher on the Healthcare Values Partnership at the Faculty of Theology and Religion, University of Oxford. She holds a DPhil in Theology and an MSt in the Study of Religion from Oxford, as well as an MA in English and Religious Studies from Aberdeen. Her research focusses on political theology, political ethics and theological perspectives on medicine, healthcare and the welfare state. In 2015, she held an award from the Saxony-Anhalt Arts Foundation to translate Richard Faber's *Political Demonology* (Wipf & Stock 2017). Therese Feiler's first monograph is entitled *Logics of War* and will be published by Bloomsbury.

Lucy Frith is Reader in Bioethics and Social Science at the University of Liverpool. Her research focusses on the social and ethical aspects of healthcare decision-making, policy and regulation. She has published widely on a range of issues in bioethics, with a long-standing interest in the social and ethical aspects of reproductive technologies.

Muir Gray published the first edition of *How To Get Better Value Healthcare* in 2007 and has been working for the NHS in England to introduce value-based healthcare to complement evidence-based healthcare, which he introduced in the 1990s. He is the director of Better Value Healthcare and a visiting professor in the University of Oxford's department of Primary Care Health Sciences. He recently launched a Masters level module in Value Based Healthcare as part of the University's new Masters level programme.

Jonathan Herring is Vice Dean and Professor of Law at the Law Faculty, Oxford University, and DM Wolfe-Clarendon Fellow in Law at Exeter College, Oxford

University. He has written on family law, medical law, criminal law and legal issues surrounding care and old age. His books include: *Vulnerable Adults and the Law* (2016); *Caring and the Law* (2014); *Older People in Law and Society* (Oxford University Press 2009); *Altruism, Welfare and the Law* (Springer 2015, with Charles Foster); *Identity, Personhood and the Law* (Springer 2017) (with Charles Foster) *European Human Rights and Family Law* (Hart 2010) (With Shazia Choudhry); *Medical Law and Ethics* (OUP 2016); *Criminal Law*, (Oxford University Press 2016); *Family Law* (Pearson 2017); and *The Woman Who Tickled Too Much* (Pearson 2009).

Joshua Hordern is Associate Professor of Christian Ethics at the Faculty of Theology and Religion in the University of Oxford and a Fellow of Harris Manchester College. His research mainly concerns how theology and religion illumine the role of affections such as compassion, joy, fear and hope in public life. Joshua Hordern leads the Oxford Healthcare Values Partnership (www.healthcarevalues.ox.ac.uk), which collaborates with healthcare bodies to improve the ethos of healthcare. He serves on the Royal College of Physicians Committee for Ethical Issues in Medicine and has received grants from the British Academy, the Wellcome Trust, the Sir Halley Stewart Trust and the Arts and Humanities Research Council. His publications include *Political Affections: Civic Participation and Moral Theology* (OUP 2013), *Compassion in Healthcare: Practical Policy for Civic Life* (OUP, forthcoming 2019) and a co-edited volume entitled *Personalised Medicine: the Promise, the Hype and the Pitfalls* (*The New Bioethics* 2017). Before coming to Oxford, he was a Research Fellow at Wolfson College, Cambridge, and a local authority councillor with St Edmundsbury Borough Council.

Ruth Horn is University Research Lecturer at the University of Oxford. She studied sociology in Germany and France and holds a PhD from the École des Hautes Études en Sciences Sociales, Paris. Her research focusses on ethical questions raised by medical practices and new technologies at the beginning and end of life. She has a particular interest in understanding the contexts (legal, cultural, socio-historical) in which ethical questions emerge, and how debates employ ethical concepts such as dignity, solidarity and autonomy. Following from her research, Ruth Horn is interested in the emotional work of professionals when dealing with distressing situations. Her previous research on advance directives in England, France and Germany was funded by the European Commission and the Wellcome Trust. Currently, she works on the Ethics Programme of the PAGE Project (Prenatal Assessment of Genomes and Exomes).

Anant Jani is Executive Director of Better Value Healthcare and a Research Fellow at the University of Oxford Value Based Healthcare Programme. He works on understanding how the key players can increase value in healthcare through greater patient involvement, healthcare systems, policy change and innovations (clinical, basic science, diagnostics, IT). Anant Jani's experience in healthcare started with his work with Sir Muir Gray in the England Department of Health

QIPP Right Care programme, where he helped localities across England design and implement high-value population-based healthcare systems. This included building the first national system for stroke prevention for patients with Atrial Fibrillation, which was a joint effort with NHS England and Public Health England. Before working in healthcare, Anant Jani was a molecular immunologist studying gene regulation and epigenetics in B- and T-cells. He completed his undergraduate studies at Brandeis University and his doctoral studies at Yale University.

Angeliki Kerasidou is Researcher in Global Health Ethics at the Ethox Centre, University of Oxford. She studied Theology and Philosophy at universities in Greece, Germany and the UK, and gained her doctorate in 2009 at Oxford University. Her research focusses on the ethics of new technologies in biomedical research and their impact in practice. She has written about the ethics of stem cell research, synthetic biology, and the ethics of genomic research, particularly in developing countries. A central theme in her work are the ethical questions that arise within professional roles (ethics and professionalism). Her current research is looking at the ways in which socio-economic changes and technological advancements are influencing the moral landscape of medical practice and research.

David Misselbrook is Associate Professor of Family Medicine at RCSI Bahrain and is Senior Ethics Adviser to the *British Journal of General Practice*. He was a General Practitioner in South London for three decades. He taught at the United Medical and Dental Schools of Guy's and St Thomas' Hospitals, and he was a GP Trainer and Course Organiser for the Lewisham General Practice Vocational Training Scheme. He taught Philosophy and Ethics for the Society of Apothecaries, was Course Director of the Society's Diploma in the Philosophy of Medicine, and serves as a past President of the Society's Faculty of the History and Philosophy of Medicine and Pharmacy. He was Dean of the Royal Society of Medicine from 2008–2011 and a member of the Directors of Continuing Professional Development Committee of the UK Academy of Medical Royal Colleges. He is the author of *Thinking about Patients* (2001), a textbook on patient-centred medicine.

Andrew Papanikitas is an Academic Clinical Lecturer in the Nuffield Department of Primary Care Health Sciences at the University of Oxford. He is a practicing medical doctor (GP) in Oxford with an academic background in history, ethics and education. His PhD thesis was entitled *From the Classroom to the Clinic: Ethics Education and General Practice*. He has taught medical ethics and law at several UK medical schools, and he has published widely on the themes of medical education and medical ethics. He is on the council of the Royal Society of Medicine GP and Primary Healthcare Section and a past President of the Open Section. He is Director for the Society of Apothecaries' Diploma Course in Philosophy and Ethics of Health Care. With John Spicer, he recently edited the *Handbook of Primary Care Ethics* (CRC Press 2017).

Pythagoras Petratos is Researcher at the Blavatnik School of Government, University of Oxford. Prior to that, he was a Departmental Lecturer in Finance at the Saïd Business School, Oxford. He holds postgraduate degrees from Cass Business School, City University, the University of London and the University of Oxford in Finance, Economics (Health), European Politics and Computer Science (Engineering) respectively. He was awarded his PhD by the University of London in 2009. He has presented at various conferences, universities and international organisations, and he is a Fellow of the Royal Society of Arts.

Adrian Walsh is a Political Philosopher at the University of New England and is interested in a wide range of philosophical and normative issues concerning economic theory, marketisation and distributive justice. He also works on questions of philosophical methodology. Walsh has been at UNE since 1997 and has taught on a diverse range of topics, including bioethics, critical reasoning, social and political philosophy, game theory, the metaphysics of personhood and philosophical method. He has held research fellowships at the University of St Andrews and the University of Helsinki and is currently an Associate Editor of the *Journal of Applied Philosophy*. He has published three books: *A neo-Aristotelian Theory of Social Justice* (1997), *Ethics, Money and Sport* (2007) and *The Morality of Money* (2008). He has recently co-edited two volumes, *The Ethical Underpinnings of Climate Economics* (2016) and *Scientific Imperialism* (2017). He is currently working on a book on 'Water and Distributive Justice.'

Foreword

The countries that developed universal health coverage in the second half of the twentieth century did so to overcome the effects of healthcare based solely on the ability to pay. They replaced the market with a state bureaucracy, funded either through tax-based systems or compulsory and regulated insurance schemes. However, the limitations of this approach are becoming increasingly obvious. No country is able to keep up with the need and demand for healthcare, resulting from population ageing and what David Eddy (1993) described as the inexorable increase in the 'volume and intensity' of medical practice: namely, the development of new technologies. Many of them fail to reduce overall costs or have created treatments for conditions that were previously untreatable.

As a consequence, marketisation has become an emerging theme in all countries, and that makes this book of vital importance for everyone involved in paying for or managing health services. It not only analyses the process of marketisation, but also considers the ethical and the moral implications of decisions that are much more profound than being based simply on an economic appraisal of options. The book is in three parts. The first part analyses the concept of marketisation from different political perspectives. The second part considers the impact of marketisation on health policy and management in a number of countries, and the third part considers the impact of marketisation on the traditional core of healthcare – the consultation between the individual clinician and the patient.

What emerges is the need for a fundamental review of the assumptions on which health service decisions are made, with the concept of a new Healthcare Covenant being proposed. This new Covenant will have to address honestly the pressures that every society will face and consider the contribution that every part of the health sector can make.

The population will continue to age, and new technologies of proven effectiveness and cost-effectiveness will emerge. What is needed is a moral and ethical framework in which the difficult decisions that every society will face can be housed. This book explores core questions about how such a framework should be conceived and what factors decision-making should take into account. It will be useful to anyone who wants to understand how marketisation's influence on healthcare's ethos and organisation have a practical impact on policies and people's lives.

Muir Gray

Eddy, D. M. (1993). Three Battles to Watch in the 1990s, JAMA 270 (4), 520–526.

Introduction

*Therese Feiler, Joshua Hordern
and Andrew Papanikitas*

This book offers an interdisciplinary collection of papers that analyse the phenomenon of marketisation in healthcare.

Why another book on marketisation? After all, grown out of the basic tenets of modernity as such, the marketisation of Western healthcare systems has now proceeded well into its fourth decade. The arguments for and against the trend go back several decades; the complaints about more and more efficiency savings, belt-tightening, and re-structuring are part and parcel of everyday medical practice – as is the language of business opportunity in medicine, hope for more health and better service, better technology and more growth.

However, the distinction between what is and what is not a market has become increasingly blurred amidst divergent discourses, policies and institutional structures. The central problem remains how to discern and assess, and how practically to encounter marketisation as a continuously developing phenomenon and concept, redefining structures, actions and characters. In addition, it is in a moment such as the present one, when the status quo is believed to be the natural norm, and when the phenomenon seems too complex to be meaningful at all, that there is a need to pause, a need to survey the situation, to examine where we are, how we got here and what is next.

In continental Europe, health services were marketised by way of administrative and structural reforms. In England, the 2012 Health and Social Care Act was widely perceived as another watershed moment in this development. This process began with business-like rationalisation measures as early as the 1960s but remains synonymous with the Thatcher era. In the U.S., both a source of marketisation impulses and a negative foil, the 2010 Affordable Care Act has become a site for contested arguments for and against marketisation. For those who are most critical of further marketisation, the battle, if not adjourned indefinitely, has been postponed to future legislative periods, has escalated into industrial action, or takes the form of healthcare workers leaving the field altogether.

Meanwhile, citizens' critique is undergoing its own kind of marketisation as the 'voice' of patient-clients, audible in social media and government policies, and it frequently replaces older, often local, and more representative forms of citizens' action such as community health councils in England. In this context, the healthcare professions are facing various threats: the marketisation of the profession (everything is a 'trade'), managerialisation (good professionalism as the 'excellent' fulfilment of efficiency-related targets), pluralisation and increased professionalisation of neighbouring tasks such as humanitarian aid. Ethics understood as a discipline dealing with individual, clinical decisions, is no doubt essential to the medical profession and curriculum here. However, the discipline may also become separated from political economy and its structures. Bioethics as the alleged 'hand-maiden' of the 'medico-industrial complex' springs to mind here. As one of the chapters will highlight, ethics itself has become a commodity for sale on the healthcare market.

All of these developments cohere with and are fuelled by technological advances, digitalisation and deregulation. These, in turn, create counter-currents such as information bubbles or over-information such as so-called 'Datix noise', the over-reporting of incidents in hospitals and hence *loss* of significant events; a desire for more 'natural', alternative medicines (and worldviews); and movements towards increasing regulation and re-nationalisation, often prompted by large-scale failure or scandal. At the same time, medical innovations such as precision medicine significantly challenge public healthcare systems by the sheer intensity of cost and demand for research resources (Feiler et al. 2017). Some form of marketisation or market thinking is often part of the response.

The present volume seeks to explore how marketisation, in its various forms, shapes and affects healthcare. With different inflections referred to as economisation, neo-liberalisation, deregulation or decentralisation, and to an extent commercialisation, the marketisation of healthcare was a paradigm shift: a shift away from, or transformation of, public, solidary or communal ideas and structures of healthcare provision towards individual health-producers and consumers as the ultimate reference point. In that sense, it is an economic as much as political, cultural and moral shift. This shift is incomplete and never straightforward. The origins and impacts of marketisation are subject to disputed historical reconstructions and easily lost under the claim that things have always been this or that way. At least in Western democracies, very few parts of any healthcare system are fully marketised, i.e. fully subject to the unconditional exchange of services based merely on supply and demand. Moreover, intricate legal systems, protective barriers and more or less subtle forms of coercion uphold the so-called free market, in healthcare and in other sectors. These, in turn, have been instituted by political decisions grounded in philosophical and theological convictions. No doubt, they vary between countries, sometimes between regions. At the same time, these deeper convictions continue to set and influence the meta-level of marketisation.

Since the volume is the result of a cross- and interdisciplinary effort, there is no advance restrictive definition of marketisation, let alone agreement on its merits or demerits. Whilst some contributors suggest the marketisation of healthcare pervasively threatens the integrity of medical practice, others are not fundamentally opposed to healthcare marketisation, but rather seek to discipline possible excesses. In order to give these differences space, the three parts of this book address marketisation in healthcare at different *formal* levels.

The first part explores contrary interpretations of 'marketisation' on a systemic level, in particular with a view to organisational-ethical formation, and with a view to the locus of ethics and medical ethics within the bigger political-economic picture. The second part presents the marketisation of healthcare at the level of health and care policy-making, discussing the ethical ramifications of specific marketisation measures. Finally, Part III examines healthcare workers' personal moral standing in a marketised healthcare system, particularly with a view to preserving and enriching compassionate care, a concern that goes deeper than, but always threatens to become, a mere political slogan.

The field of medicine, markets, and ethics often shies away from addressing the systemic, intellectually comprehensive significance of particular cases or policies. Equally, it is difficult to trace the policy-effects of ideas driving systemic shifts. Hence, another aim is to break through the barrier between empirical and normative that runs through research on the ethics of healthcare and medicine in a marketised system. Additionally, as we intentionally obfuscate the artificial borderline between 'hard' and 'soft' disciplines, the present volume takes an important step towards a richer, more sophisticated and discerning public reflection on the implications of marketised healthcare systems, and perhaps public welfare in general. Concepts such as 'the market', 'the common good', 'compassion', 'representation', 'wellbeing', etc. require concrete definitions and substantive debate. In particular, as the need for 'holistic' care in the NHS is increasingly promoted, the humanities play a key role in unpacking what that might mean. They are able to save these terms both from becoming 'magic concepts' (Pollitt and Hupe 2011) that can mean anything, and from becoming phrases without meaning that make no difference to either healthcare workers' or patients' self-understanding and behaviour.

Hence, each part of the book follows a distinct format that seeks to unpack conceptually how marketisation works. Crucially, rather than presenting a unified solution, theoretical viewpoints will be productively contrasted. The significance of these juxtapositions emerge in concrete examples, whether within the approaches offered or in conversations between chapters. Finally, synthesising chapters in each part to some extent constructively summarises and/or creatively takes forward the material covered in the immediately preceding chapters.

As the contributors reflect on the meaning and influence of marketisation in its fourth decade, the aim is to identify viable possibilities of integrity in healthcare today. Again, rather than indulging in a woolly consensus or mere diversity, the aim has been to demarcate current fault lines of the debate and to search for sharper clarity in a field with an ambiguous plurality of discourses. The collection as a whole and the interaction between its parts aims to support practical reasoning by reflecting on the historical roots of marketisation, alongside its political, cultural and philosophical underpinnings and existing practical manifestations.

1. Part I

Part I of the book, 'The place of the market', introduces marketisation as a systemic phenomenon. Pythagoras Petratos, writing from the perspective of Hayekian economics, opens this section. This approach has been the leading and contested thought-frame for marketisation since the first half of the twentieth century.

Petratos makes the case for decentralisation of healthcare – and thus a form of marketisation. His reference point is the economic calculation debate. The debate revolves around the level of centralisation in socialist and capitalist systems, highlighting the need for a pricing mechanism to determine the value of goods and services. Petratos introduces Ludwig von Mises, Friedrich von Hayek, and the Polish economist Oskar R. Lange, all of whom to various degrees critiqued full-scale central planning with a view to the Soviet Union. The historical background is central to understanding not least why marketisation continues to be associated with an element of liberation. In terms of ethics, Petratos embraces classic and preference utilitarianism. Importantly, despite (or because of) this stance, he restricts the concern of economics from the outset. He separates it from what he refers to as *political* questions: distribution and justice, as well as the concrete forms authorities governing healthcare might take. In the second part of his chapter, Petratos then highlights the need and difficulty in classifying healthcare systems so as to assess them economically and map them on the spectrum of the economic calculation between centralisation and marketisation.

The following chapter marks a stark counter-point to Petratos' view. Miran Epstein, speaking from a medical and Marxist point of view, begins with what he calls the 'ostensible paradox': present day 'patient-centred' medicine abuses both patients and doctors precisely when it follows its own ethic to the letter. Against several ways to explain this paradox away – some of which are endorsed later in this volume – he argues that the ethic itself is merely a result of irreconcilable conflicts of material interest. It is a compromise and ideological superstructure that allows the forces of Capital to perpetuate their supremacy and extract abnormal profits whilst falsely appearing as 'ethical medicine'. Epstein then argues that in order to have a truly humanist ethic – as opposed to a misanthropic ethic – an ethic that serves doctors and patients, we first need humanist material conditions. Interestingly, Epstein separates the unearthing of the irreconcilable conflict that led to the 'ethical' compromise as a historical task that is distinct from questions of moral justification. This historical materialism – with the aim of liberation – puts him in closer proximity to Petratos than it might seem at first. Nonetheless, these two approaches continue to represent two diametrically opposed political-economic positions underlying healthcare in the West: one utilitarian-economist, the other critical-humanist.

In the final chapter of the section, Lucy Frith presents a possible mediate path between Petratos and Epstein, developing it with a view to the English National Health Service (NHS). As mentioned above, the 2012 Health and Social Care Act presents a major push for the marketisation of the NHS. It includes decentralised responsibilities, more space for commercial companies and social enterprises, as well as competition. Frith here highlights a range of problems that this has created. The contradiction of the state 'buying' and contracting healthcare, whilst the patient is supposedly a freely choosing consumer should not go unmentioned. Frith also notes the recent moves away from marketisation in reaction to such problems. Drawing on Illich and Epstein, she then develops an argument for organisational ethics, an extension of bioethics that is both close to the organisation and yet refuses the role of an institutional handmaiden or mere psychological buffer. Organisational ethics would arise out of professional obligations, legal structures and NHS foundational principles, but also involve community stakeholders. Frith's chapter thus explores the grounds for a new emancipatory politics between the entrenched or conciliatory forums within marketised healthcare organisations on the one hand, and the formerly central political authorities at the national level on the other.

2. Part II

Part II, 'The influence of the market', looks at the effects of marketisation on policy, whilst in preparation for Part III it keeps in mind the moral formation of healthcare workers. This section asks, "how does marketisation influence the practical structures of healthcare?" At the level of policy, the moral significance of marketisation will be explored illustratively through health-economic encodings such as Diagnosis-Related Groups (DRGs)., the introduction of personal care budgets and litigation avoidance or 'defensive medicine'. Therese Feiler challenges the marketisation discourse from a religious-philosophical perspective. She examines an influential measure operationalising marketisation worldwide at the meso-level: DRGs. These groups demonstrate the underlying assumptions of marketisation: a philosophical and religious neutrality (to an extent put forth in Part I of this volume); marketisation as an evolutionary process in the face of economic necessities; the claim that care is now better represented and more efficiently accounted for; and finally that marketisation does not touch the substance of medicine. Feiler sets four theologically informed counter-points against these assumptions. Echoing Epstein, she exposes marketisation as a comprehensive 'transvaluation' of healthcare that needs to be contrasted with a more fundamental reality of givenness and gift. Second, marketisation needs to be confronted with its own history. This is central to reintegrate healthcare 'policy' into political negotiations, and hence to assert political responsibility over against impersonal processes. Third, Feiler points at the distortions of health-economic codifications, arguing that representations of care need to follow rather than blot out the care actually given. Finally, she posits a transformative vocation against the clash of medical and economic logics experienced by many doctors, nurses and therapists.

In a comparably critical way, Jonathan Herring presents a shift towards personal budgets as a new approach of the state to social care in England. Rather than the local authority providing services and equipment to meet someone's care needs, the person in need is now given a budget that they can use to purchase the required services. The services may be purchased from the local authority or other providers. The aim is to put people in charge of determining how to meet their care needs. Herring regards personal budgets as an expression of consumerist personal autonomy. Moreover, in order to be effective, consumerism relies on the market responding to improve quality and reduce cost. He argues that a reliance on consumerism in this instance is based on a false view of autonomy and fails to adequately appreciate the nature of care. Good care, Herring points out, is not about independence but interdependence. It is not about empowering, but sharing vulnerabilities. Good care is not about self-determination, but a mutual sharing of our relational autonomies. Care cannot be packaged, valued or budgeted. In its nature, it is relational, involving responsibilities and the intermingling of interests and identities. Care is something we all do and we all need; it is not placing a burden on others. Our social interventions need to rejoice in care, enable and support it, Herring argues. The idea of care as a marketised package is an altogether negligent starting point.

Anant Jani and Andrew Papanikitas examine defensive medicine as a markets-related phenomenon that has increasing prevalence across healthcare systems globally. They divide defensive medicine into two broad categories: positive defensive medicine, or assurance behaviour, occurs when unnecessary services (i.e. diagnostic tests, procedures, referrals) are provided to patients to reduce the chance of patients taking legal action against a physician; negative defensive medicine, or avoidance behaviour, occurs when physicians refuse to provide risky procedures and/or provide care to high risk patients. Defensive medicine, they argue, increases the financial costs of healthcare delivery, decreases the quality and safety of healthcare and reduces access to healthcare – it harms both justice in healthcare delivery and the markets themselves. The authors consider how defensive medicine both influences and is influenced by a healthcare market and provide some of the proposed solutions. Jani and Papanikitas note that the factors that could lead healthcare to operate as a 'true and rational' market (and as a result to increase its quality, safety and value) are the same factors that are driving defensive medicine. Healthcare markets, they suggest, need to account for irrational self-interest both on the part of the healthcare user and the healthcare professional. The key understandings of the situation have important implications for how the healthcare community might work together to utilise these factors to facilitate, rather than hinder, healthcare system improvement.

Joshua Hordern's pastoral-theological approach brings a critical synthesis to Part II and builds bridges to Parts I and III of the book. Hordern argues that covenantal thought and practice has the capacity to discipline marketisation processes in service of an ethos of gracious compassion in healthcare. He engages critically with the analyses of Diagnosis-Related Groups, Personal Budgets and defensive medicine offered by Feiler, Herring, Jani and Papanikitas in the preceding three chapters, showing that the key themes of 'care' and 'work' can be illumined by a covenantal approach which works judiciously with healthcare marketisation. Constructively, Hordern draws on parallels in the Armed Services to argue for five markers of a written and institutionalised Healthcare Covenant between health and care workers and the public. Drawing on traditions of pastoral and political theology to explore the psychological and social influences of marketisation, this chapter provides the bridge between the systemic issues of Part I, the policy concerns of Part II and the questions of professional ethics considered in Part III.

3. Part III

The third part of the volume will problematise the place of professionals in a marketised healthcare system, juxtaposing different in-roads into medical ethics. This sets a new tone as far as the general unease with marketisation usually relies on moral intuitions that cannot be taken for granted. Therefore, this section starts with an examination of the ends of commercialisation, with a particular eye on the Australian experience of marketisation. In his chapter, the philosopher Adrian Walsh develops what he calls the Corrosion Thesis. Against a socialist abolitionism of commercialisation and a capitalist full-scale endorsement – both encountered in Part I of the volume – Walsh argues that the market presents health professionals with various moral *hazards* which threaten to corrode medical ideals. As significant risks, they require vigilance on the part of health professionals and legislation to restrict the possibilities of behaviour in which the pursuit of profit overshadows significant moral values. Drawing in particular on the Kantian objection against commodification of human beings as ends-in-themselves, Walsh presents arguments for rejecting a commercialisation of healthcare while recognising some of its merits, as highlighted by Petratos in Chapter 1.

David Misselbrook, himself a practitioner of and lecturer in medicine, transposes Walsh's considerations into Aristotelian virtue ethics and asks what it actually means to be a virtuous professional amidst processes of marketisation. The prime loci of moral concern for him are the communities of medical practice and their traditions reaching back to Hippocrates. According to Misselbrook, they draw their culture both from moral theory and from the marketplace. In that sense, he somewhat echoes Frith's and Hordern's perspectives. If healthcare is to pursue the proper goals of medicine, he argues, the turn to a capitalist market-narrative is morally problematic. Notions of human flourishing, which gives particular priority to the weak and vulnerable, are ill-adapted to a market narrative that sees no problem in the strong dominating the weak. The virtuous practitioner, however, will pursue the *telos* of medicine rather than market forces. This *telos*, Misselbrook argues, will be achieved as professionals practice compassion and wisdom, whilst paying attention to the *polis* or social environment of healthcare.

The recent emphasis on empathy, particularly the measurability of its conditions, has been an important way to newly criticise the corrosive dimensions and tenets of marketisation and commercialisation. Angeliki Kerasidou's and Ruth Horn's chapter engages with the notion of empathy both in solidaristic and private healthcare systems. The authors, combining philosophical and sociological expertise, suggest that for care to be empathetic not just selectively, the individual professional's efforts alone are not enough. The professional code teaches doctors and nurses to engage empathetically with their patients, but the demand cannot be fully met in private, i.e. market-based, healthcare systems, which operate on the principle of optimising self-interest. Instead, Kerasidou and Horn argue, the healthcare system as a whole needs to embrace empathy as one of its principles and make it the basis on which it operates. Ensuring empathetic care for all can be better achieved in a system that acknowledges people's interdependency and mutual responsibilities, as in a public system. Hence, instead of putting the moral onus on professionals, the authors insist that a systemic shift allowing for empathy is indispensable. This partly overlaps with Feiler's insistence on the healthcare system as an object of political responsibility, in contrast to the market's and marketeers' problematic focusses on the single patient or doctor.

Andrew Papanikitas picks up the challenge set by Walsh and Misselbook. He suggests that any form of market presents ethical issues for healthcare professionals – these are issues that are both related and unrelated to the economic drivers of healthcare. His inference is that these are best navigated with sound policy, good education and healthcare environments that meaningfully support ethical practice. These, he suggests, can be framed as a market in healthcare ethics. He discusses current and possible forms of a market in healthcare ethics which serves a wider healthcare sector, noting that those who offer research and education in healthcare ethics are as subject to market forces as providers of healthcare. Echoing Kerasidou and Horn, he argues that a market in healthcare ethics – if it is to serve effectively a broader healthcare market and society – must sustain 'everyday' aspects of good healthcare. If it concentrates primarily on policy or on novel technologies, it will only offer a partial good. Whether or not ethics ought to be commodified – he argues that, unless it is appropriately resourced, pressures to concentrate on paid activities in a healthcare market will mean that healthcare ethics research is shaped by whoever is prepared to pay for it, and healthcare ethics education will be haphazardly provided – for a market in healthcare ethics to work, purchasers must recognise value in healthcare ethics activities, and providers must offer products that are meaningful to purchasers. He calls for further research into healthcare ethics as a market.

4. Advancing the debate

With this volume, we aim to advance the debate on marketisation towards new ways of creative, critical analysis by identifying and charting pathways towards compassionate healthcare. Self-reflectively debating the nature, place and role of ethics as such continues to be a task, as it prevents ethics from becoming a mere moralisation of the status quo or a tool for corporate white-washing. Interdisciplinary engagement continues to prompt methodological reflections, e.g. on the limitations of scientific paradigms to grasp what is at stake in healthcare, or the possibilities of identifying moral or normative tendencies and conceptual pitfalls long before empirical research becomes available. Policy-makers increasingly implement measures – organisational structures, regulations – according to the principle of trial-and-error. However, patients and healthcare workers are too vulnerable to be exposed to experimental policy-making devoid of conceptual and moral sense. Hence, there is a renewed need for conceptual clarity, for insight into the moral nature of organisational structures and the foreseeable impacts of policy on the delicate cultural-moral ecology of healthcare.

References

Feiler, T., Gaitskell, K., Maughan, T., and Hordern, J. (eds.) (2017). Personalised Medicine: The Promise, the Hype and the Pitfalls. *The New Bioethics*, 23 (1), Special Issue.

Pollitt, C. and Hupe, P. (2011). Talking about Government: The Role of Magic Concepts, *Public Management Review*, 13 (5), 641–658.

Online resources

Interviews, lectures, short articles, and even a simulated debate on healthcare between pre-deceased philosophers 'John Rawls' and 'Robert Nozick' are available at the website of the University of Oxford Healthcare Values Partnership: www.healthcarevalues.ox.ac. uk/marketisation-ethics-and-healthcare-0

Part I
The place of the market

1 Why the economic calculation debate matters

The case for decentralisation in healthcare

Pythagoras Petratos

Introduction

A major concern in healthcare is its rising cost. As the economic burden of health-care is increasing, there is greater focus on the efficiency of healthcare systems. One of the major debates in economic history about efficiency is the *'Economic Calculation Problem'*. The economic calculation problem mainly regards the level of centralisation of economic systems. In general, the argument is that decen-tralised systems, featuring market mechanisms, are more efficient in allocating resources. The economic calculation problem has many dimensions and aspects, some of which I will discuss below. However, the main argument of this chapter will be that healthcare flourishes best in a decentralised system.

An important dimension of decentralisation and market forces in healthcare systems concerns ethics. Ethics in this context is often understood as the discipline concerned with individual and clinical decisions. However, ethics in its broader sense may also include the political economy of healthcare. In that sense, this paper attempts to shed light on a less well-researched field, the application of eco-nomic theory to healthcare. The main argument – that better healthcare is attained in decentralised systems – is framed in utilitarian terms. In order to bridge ethics with economics, a *consequentialist* perspective is adopted. The moral objective is to maximise utility, and more precisely the utility associated with health. This is based on fundamental principles of *classic utilitarianism*. Its proponent Jeremy Bentham (1789) put great emphasis on the 'pleasure of health' among the vari-ous pleasures and pains. Hence, classic utilitarianism enables us to account for additional utilitarian "pleasures" and value beyond the rather narrow sense of economic units. The discipline of economic evaluation in healthcare analyses some of the limitations and methodologies used in order to represent utility in health in terms of monetary units. Nevertheless, the expression of utility in monetary terms remains the most popular method in economic evaluation in healthcare, since costs are always captured in economic units and benefits (i.e. cost-benefit analysis).[1]

Another moral principle is the fulfillment of individual preferences. *Preference utilitarianism* is considered to be a critical part of healthcare. This is because a lack of health involves suffering and pain, which is frequently a matter of individual tolerance. Moreover, many health conditions involve individual lifestyles, risk attitudes, and in general a wide range of individual preferences and subjective valuations that, I argue, should be freely expressed. At this point, it might be useful to clarify the meaning and conditions of choice. We should consider choice to be free of any coercion. The position of this paper is that competition and therefore pluralism in choice should be encouraged and achieved.

The economic calculation problem is widely known for its influence on political and organisational science. Because of this extension into other fields, it has also been identified as the *'Socialist Calculation Debate'*. However, it should be emphasised from the beginning that the economic problem needs to be split from its political aspects. The focus in this chapter is on cost-efficiency and utilitarian arguments rather than distribution or other political issues. In that sense, the question of distribution is regarded as an exclusively political rather than economic issue. This is in accordance with Ludwig von Mises (1920), a key figure in the Socialist Calculation debate, who states that 'distribution of consumption goods must be independent of the question of production and its economic conditions'.

Hence, the present analysis will focus on economic efficiency: which economic conditions can produce more, or ideally, a maximum of both wealth and health? Mises acknowledges that this requires the appointment of a special body to manage production, appointed by a political process. This can be a dictatorship or a democratically elected government. And of course, the political process is very important. Nevertheless, following again Mises' argument, the perspective in this essay remains purely economic.

Importantly, in the context of the original debate, 'socialist system' is used here in a specific sense. 'Under Socialism all the means of production are the property of the community. It is the community alone that can dispose of them and which determines their use of production' (Mises 1920). Socialism in this context is synonymous with communism. This is quite different from today's perception of socialism, which is often considered to be a mixed economy of social democracy.

Market failures and externalities are additional economic issues to which we should pay attention. Market failures are situations in which the allocation of economic resources is not efficient, due to asymmetric information, irrational behaviour, and a lack of competition. External effects (externalities) occur when an individual's actions affect another who did not choose to incur this economic effect. In healthcare, there can be many types of market failures and externalities. However, for reasons of space and simplicity the discussion of market failures and externalities will be excluded here. Nevertheless, competition and information remain key themes. Another term to clarify in advance is the notion of 'profit'. Normal profit is often confused with abnormal profits. The former represents the reward of labourers or entrepreneurs for their work and risky undertakings. The latter occurs in cases where market failures prevail and individuals or enterprises can extract economic rents resulting in excess profits. The focus here is on normal profits.

The following discussion is divided into three main sections. The first section critically reviews the history and evolution of the economic calculation debate. The historical progress of the original Mises-Hayek argument is discussed as well as the Lange-Lerner model. The second section examines the structure of different healthcare systems and assesses if, and to what extent, the economic calculation problem applies to them. The UK National Health Service (NHS) represents the main reference case. The final section will summarise the previous sections and suggest how decentralised markets can contribute towards more affordable and better quality healthcare.

1. The history and evolution of the economic calculation problem

1.1 Economic calculation in the socialist commonwealth – Ludwig von Mises

We have already noted that the economic calculation debate started with Ludwig von Mises (1920). Arguably, this debate can even be identified with the so-called Mises-Hayek critique of central planning (Meadowcroft 2003). While there are suggestions of profound differences between Mises and Hayek, these differences are small when compared to the rest of economic thought in the twentieth century (Boettke 1998). Our intention here is to first present the arguments of Ludwig von Mises and then analyse the positions of Friedrich von Hayek, the 1974 Nobel Laureate in Economics. We will then have a complete overview of the original and complete Mises-Hayek critique.

Mises (1920) mainly wrote his critique during a time when socialist parties were gaining power in Russia, Hungary, Austria and other countries, and different types of socialist systems were evolving. The prevailing ideology was Marxism, as the Bolsheviks had taken over and were consolidating their power in Russia. Mises (1920, p. 38) concluded that Marxist writers preferred to focus on the immediate future and the 'path to Socialism and not Socialism itself' – 'they are not even conscious of the larger problem of economic calculation in a socialist society'.

So Mises was writing with highly, or even totally centralised economies in view. The final step to a socialist nationalisation programme, according to the Austrian Marxist Otto Bauer, is the socialisation of banks and their amalgamation into a single central bank, of which the administrative board would be the 'supreme economic authority, the chief administrative organ of the whole society' (Mises 1920, p. 39). Part of Mises' critique (1920) is that in the case of a single centralised bank, the monetary system as it was known would disappear, and there would be problems with credit.

Although central banking and monetary policy are not key concerns in the context of healthcare, they have broader economic implications for our analysis. First, without an effective monetary policy inflation rises, which has consequences for every aspect of economic life, including healthcare. Second, the availability of credit and the financing function has effects on how much money can be allocated to the healthcare system. Third, an effective monetary policy is critical in healthcare to finance entrepreneurship and innovation in order to find new cures for illnesses or improve existing ones.

Every person makes some *value judgment* in order to choose between the satisfaction of one need against another (Mises 1920). This value judgement is basically utilitarian because the person intends to satisfy their individual needs. A rational individual would be able to appropriately value goods of lower or higher utility order. 'But where the state of affairs is more involved and their interconnections not so easily discernible, subtler means must be employed to accomplish a correct valuation of the means of production' (Mises 1920, p. 8).

According to Mises, in order to attain a correct valuation and optimise production, an exchange economy is necessary. It is then possible to make a calculation that entails the valuation of all participants in the trade. An exchange economy is also an inclusive mechanism that respects and accounts for all participants' preferences. No one can be excluded, and therefore it can be viewed as a democratic process in which every individual participates in a process to determine the price. Access is not fundamentally limited in the exchange process. Every individual can participate. Even absence from the exchange can be regarded as non-active participation, since it affects demand for healthcare services, and thus monetary values (prices).

Participants can value the goods according to their preferences and at the same time calculate how much of their own labour is required in order to attain or produce them.

> Anyone who wishes to make calculations in regard to a complicated process of production will immediately notice whether he has worked more economically than others or not; if he finds from reference to the exchange relations obtaining in the market, that he will not be able to produce profitably.
>
> (Mises 1920, p. 10)

Another advantage is that individuals can easily refer to monetary – in this case, values – and connect them to utility. Since goods are substitutes for each other in accordance with the exchange relations, the participant can use the monetary value as a guide to choosing which goods to obtain. This is the basic line of Mises' argument regarding the benefits of the market exchange. The process of production is even more complicated regarding a plant or a large energy project because 'vague valuations' cannot be applied.

In his early work, Mises is more concerned with the economic mechanism, although in later works he focusses more on the importance of choice (e.g. *Human Action* 1940). As stated in the introduction above, the perspective here is classic and preference utilitarianism. An important conclusion from the brief analysis of Mises' critique is that everyone can choose freely. In socialism, by contrast, it is the central committee or other types of centralised authority which make decisions. These decisions most likely do not represent individual needs and preferences. At this point, it is useful to mention that choice depends on the degree of centralisation and administration. We can say that Mises was prophetic about what would happen in Russia. In 1921, the State Planning Committee, known as Gosplan, was established, and the main line of Mises' arguments stems from this very centralisation of decision-making. Eventually communism in Russia collapsed.

In the former U.S.S.R., which is probably the example closest to socialism as theorised by Mises, decision-making was highly centralised and centrally controlled through the Soviet Health Ministry in Moscow. It 'controls health care facilities, medical education training, personnel, and financial resources throughout the Soviet Union'. (Rowland and Telyukov 1991, p. 76). Medical personnel were appointed by the Ministry and did not have much choice of where to go or what to do. Plenty of anecdotal evidence exists about healthcare in the U.S.S.R. Physicians' salaries were approximately 75% of the average per capita income (Friedenberg 1987), And there were local health boards administering the healthcare services in different regions. Although in theory these were considered to be the voice of the people and to represent their choices, in practice, the boards were just passive intermediaries in the distribution of funds from the Ministry to the local health service providers (Rowland and Telyukov 1991). Thus, patients did not have much choice and in general, the quality of the services was inferior to that of the U.S. and numerous other capitalist economies. I will examine later the idiosyncrasies of different healthcare systems with regard to choice.

According to Mises, the second conclusion to be drawn from the inferiority of centralised planning (and healthcare), is that socialist systems are inefficient and it is 'impossible' for them to survive. He pays significant attention to the competitive forces of an exchange. This is in accord with basic economic laws, such as the law that a competitive equilibrium is Pareto optimal. Named after the Vilfredo Pareto (1848–1923), a prominent contributor to welfare economics, Pareto optimal is a condition in which resources are allocated in such a way that an individual or preference cannot be any better off, without making another individual worse off. In contrast, a socialist system is not only a monopoly but also most critically in this context, a monopsony. It does not allow choice and participation in an exchange. Consequently, it does not facilitate any competition or wealth creation. Therefore, socialism in its original form violates the classic utilitarian principle of utility maximisation.

1.2 Friedrich von Hayek and the Mises-Hayek critique

Friedrich von Hayek, a colleague of von Mises in Austria and later winner of the Nobel Prize in Economics, significantly advanced the argument against central planning. Hayek (1935), revising the nature and history of the socialist calculation debate, observed that it had been reduced to only a problem of 'psychology and education'. Thus, it was considered by many to be a mere problem of value judgements: people agreeing or disagreeing with it was seen as a problem of ethics. Hayek (1935) also criticised a widespread belief that economic problems do not exist in a socialist world; in his view, people who hold these opinions often do not understand economic problems.

Hayek identifies the essential point in Mises work: that pricing was to be applied to all intermediary levels and factors of production; no other process but the pricing mechanism in a competitive market could account for all the facts (Hayek 1935). At approximately the same time, two other notable studies appeared. The sociologist Max Weber (1921) also argued that economic problems cannot be solved in a rational manner by socialist systems. The main conclusion of the distinguished Russian economist Boris Brutzkus had many similarities with the work of Mises and Weber (Hayek 1935). Of interest is not only this conclusion, but also the fact that his work contains direct empirical observations from inside the U.S.S.R. It can also be regarded as the first Russian critique of socialism. Brutzkus was almost immediately exiled from the U.S.S.R., and that is the reason his writings became known only much later (Brutzkus 1921).

Hayek (1935) elaborates on the difference between engineering and determinism on the one hand, and the very different character of the economic problem and *in natura* calculations on the other. The engineer is faced with fixed conditions when calculating how much steel or how many labourers are required to complete a project. These are mainly technological problems. However, economic decision-making cannot be made with an absolute process, as in engineering. Economic problems arise as soon as different purposes compete for these limited resources (Hayek 1935). It would be hard or even impossible for a central planner to make such a decision without prices. Without prices, there would just be the subjective decision of the central planner. This would likely not represent the preferences of the population. Thus, central decision-making would be arbitrary and lack accountability.

Hayek (1935, p. 7) uses an example particularly relevant to healthcare,

> It may well be that the need for one additional doctor is greater than the need for one additional teacher, yet under conditions where it costs three times as much to train an additional doctor than it costs to train an additional school teacher, three additional school teachers may appear preferable to one doctor.

This marginal utility trade-off can be generalised for healthcare services. Would we prefer one more doctor to three more nurses or five more physiotherapists, or more surgeons than ophthalmologists, or more geriatric services than pediatric services? Hence, prices and values are essential when making meaningful decisions, and without them choices can seem completely arbitrary.

By 1940, Hayek considered that some of the issues around the economics of socialism had been solved. First, economists had accepted that socialism could not dispense with value and monetary calculations and replace them with any other units *in natura*. Second, economists had rejected the proposal that values, rather than being left to be determined by competition, can be calculated by central planners using mathematical economics. Hayek quotes Pareto saying that even with a system of simultaneous equations, 'if one really could know all these equations, the only available means to solve them is to observe the practical solution given by the market' (Hayek 1940, p. 126). In other words, the market offered a means to reduce complexity and arbitrariness in decision-making.

The real question about the application of competitive principles to a socialist society 'was not whether they ought to apply, but whether they could in practice be applied in the absence of a market' (Hayek 1940, p. 127). Hayek wonders how competition could fit in with the purpose of a socialist system; after all, competition and central planning were considered opposites. An additional criticism of Hayek regards the arbitrary character of the initial form and values of a fixed price system as proposed by Oskar R. Lange and Henry Douglas Dickinson. Starting with an inefficient economic disequilibrium, Hayek argued, could result in significant welfare losses reducing overall wealth and, effectively, health.

Hayek's second criticism concerns the time that Lange's hypothesis might take to obtain a proper solution by trial and error. Hayek (1940, pp. 131–132) argues that in the real world, the rules are of the continuous change of economic data, and he suggests that

> Whether and how far anything approaching the desirable equilibrium is ever reached depends entirely on the speed with which the adjustment can be made. The practical problem is not whether a particular method would eventually lead to a hypothetical equilibrium, but which method will secure the more rapid and complete adjustment to the daily changing conditions in different places and different industries.

So not only is there a welfare loss due to the disequilibrium, but this disequilibrium is also dynamic and constantly changing. A fixed price mechanism, as in a socialist system, cannot adjust quickly enough to continuously changing conditions. This can result in a substantial reduction of utility.

Moreover, Hayek (1940) points to some practical applications of competition in socialist systems. Although fixing prices may be justified for some standardised, rarely changing commodities, the situation is different with commodities that cannot be standardised and are produced daily, often to individual orders. Finally, he proceeds to discuss the complications of calculations in a socialist system and how the role of the entrepreneur can be taken away by the central authority. This can result in a reduction of innovations therefore preventing the invention of more efficient technologies and new therapies.

One of the most significant contributions of Hayek is his work on the use of knowledge and the importance of information in decision-making and choices. In order to construct a rational economic order, the fundamental question that concerns Hayek (1945) is: What is the actual problem that needs solving by the market? The answer is the possession of all relevant information and a system of preferences; 'how to secure the best knowledge to any of the members of the society' (1945). Hayek (1945) also stresses that economic problems arise as consequences of changes in conditions, and that day-to-day adjustments are important. This point is especially critical in the twenty-first century, where technologies are disruptively and increasingly changing. Modern healthcare is also subject to major and continuous technological changes.

> We cannot expect that this problem will be solved by first communicating all this knowledge to a central board which, after integrating *all* knowledge,

issues its orders. We must solve it by some form of decentralisation . . . [to] ensure that the knowledge of the particular circumstances and place will be promptly used.

(Hayek 1945, p. 524)

While it is impossible for a central planning authority to acquire all this knowledge, prices can reflect the preferences and actions of different people on the ground. Hence, prices provide the mechanism for the adjustment to changing conditions. Pricing is the most efficient mechanism since all the information about global conditions can be incorporated in real time. 'We must look at the price system as such a mechanism for communicating information, if we want to understand its real function' (Hayek 1945).

1.3 Oskar Lange and competition in socialism

We have presented much of the Mises-Hayek critique applied to socialism, but it would be a big omission not to mention the prominent contribution of the Polish economist and diplomat Oskar Lange. Lange's work, most notably *On the Economic Theory of Socialism*, can be regarded as revolutionary. His model later became known as market socialism, or the 'Third Way'. It departed from numerous Marxist assumptions and reduced the level of central planning. Lange (1936) recognised the extraordinary contribution of Mises, saying that his statue 'ought to occupy an honourable place in the great hall of the Ministry of Socialisation or of the Central Planning Board of the socialist state.' For Lange, Mises' critique forced the socialists to accept the importance of a system of economic accounting to allocate resources.

Lange (1936) recognised that a major economic problem is that of choice. He bases his argument on three notions: preferences; the knowledge about alternatives on offer; and knowledge about the resource amounts. Preferences and knowledge of resources are available to central planners, 'by the demand schedules of individuals, or can be established by the judgement of the authorities administering the economic system' (Lange 1936, p. 62). However, as we already heard, central planning authorities' judgment can be completely arbitrary, inaccurate and therefore inefficient. However, Lange's observation of the demand functions is an interesting point since they can actually reveal preferences. He also argues that availability and information about resources can be defined by production functions.

The main point of contention, according to Lange, is the knowledge of alternatives, and he constructs a model of a competitive market administered by trial and error. We should regard it as a sophisticated model with many market assumptions. Freedom of choice in consumption and freedom of choice in occupation are assumed. This is a major departure from rigid central planning. Lange (1936) recognised that some important parts of this model are arbitrary, such as the rate, or the speed, of capital accumulation. He comments that this might result in diminishing welfare and it can only be solved if capital accumulation is left to individual savings. However, he concedes, there are political limitations imposed by the socialist system that would not allow that (Lange 1945). Hence, the model as proposed by Lange has welfare constraints and thus does not maximise utility.

Market socialism offers a very different alternative to socialism as proposed by Marxists and other early proponents. Lange understood how critical the economic problem was in socialist theory and how it was neglected. His seminal contribution made Hayek (1940, p. 129) wonder, 'why he refuses to go the whole hog and to restore the price mechanism in full'. From a preference-utilitarian perspective, Lange's proposal offers free choice to individuals regarding their occupation and consumption. In that sense, it fulfils ethical considerations similar to those in free markets. Nevertheless, considerable constraints regarding choice, such as choosing to accumulate capital, remain. Consequently, some of these limitations, as well as other deadweight loss problems, do not facilitate utility maximisation in a Paretian sense, i.e. in such a way that an individual or preference cannot be any better off without making another individual worst off. Although Lange's model is a significant improvement on earlier socialism, it could not attain the level of choice and utility reached in decentralised markets.

2. Healthcare systems around the world: types, classification and centralisation

Healthcare systems can be assumed to reflect the characteristics of the broader economy with respect to the economic calculation debate discussed in the previous section. The following is an initial examination of the different types of healthcare systems in this context. The purpose of this section is to identify the dimensions of various healthcare system typologies that are relevant to central planning. The main proposition is that decentralised healthcare systems better promote healthcare utility and choice. The classification of healthcare systems facilitates the examination of their performance and therefore the maximisation of utility. Moreover, it facilitates the assessment of which healthcare systems and constituent factors allow more choice to individuals. Studies on healthcare systems have not achieved a coherent and robust conceptual framework for conducting comparative analysis and consequently there are various categorisations (Wendt et al. 2009). However, a common denominator in these classifications remains the distinction between state and private dimensions of healthcare systems. This can be a parallelism to socialist/centralised and market/decentralised systems respectively.

Notable distinctions are between public and private financing, provision and general access (Bambra 2005). An early study by Field (1973) used a typology that included, on the one side, a socialised health system in which all healthcare facilities and services are owned and controlled by the state, and on the other side, a pluralist health system with private service provision and doctors' autonomy. An OECD typology identifies three main types of healthcare system: the national health service model, owned and administered by the state and funded by general taxes; the social insurance model, with universal coverage funded by social contribution but with the capacity for the private provision of services; and finally, the private insurance model, in which financing, services, and ownership are private (OECD 1987). Later studies (Blank and Burau 2004; Giaimo and Manow 1999; Moran 1999) used similar classifications based on the state – private dichotomy.

Another classification that accounts for both public and private elements, as well as additional important healthcare parameters, was developed by Wendt et al. (2009). It could be argued that it has many similarities with previous studies, but it has a more extensive character. They identify three ideal types across the field of healthcare, namely *state healthcare systems, societal,* and finally *private healthcare systems.* This framework also contains three main aspects of healthcare: funding, provision, and regulation. In this way, 27 classes of healthcare systems are generated according to the level of state intervention or private initiative in each dimension. Wendt et al. (2009) assume that one dimension does not necessarily determine the others, and dimensions might not be uniform and rank healthcare systems according to particular sets of actors and institutions.

This is reflected in the subcategories of many cases of mixed type systems – state, societal, private, and *pure mixed.* This additional subcategory (pure mixed) expresses dimensions that are not like any others in ideal type classes. In that sense, the classification framework allows for extra flexibility if a dimension does not fall within the limits of ideal types. From the Hayek-Mises perspective adopted in this chapter, the great value of this model, despite the extended number of categories, is that it depicts the pure mixed type. It offers a rather dynamic perspective from which to assess and classify the spectrum of healthcare systems that fit the traditional categories, can be subject to continuous changes, or can be too complex to categorise.

The *World Health Report 2000,* published by the World Health Organisation (WHO), can be considered a major breakthrough in the assessment of healthcare systems' performance. This report clarifies and quantifies goals of healthcare systems and relates them to factors that contribute to them. It is therefore interesting to briefly look at the *criteria* used to describe and rank the world's healthcare systems, *and observe their relevance and influence on the economic calculation debate.* An interesting part of the report is the examination of the structure of health system financing and provision. The report presents four factors: revenue collection, pooling, purchasing, and provision, and it often assesses them in relation to government involvement and private enterprise.

The first observation is that these factors vary substantially among healthcare systems in different countries. In Table 1.1 we can see some of these differences. The NHS is a highly centralised system that is funded mainly by general taxation and social insurance, while private insurance and out of pocket play a very small role in financing. In the same fashion, the NHS is equally dominated by government administration through the Department of Health (DoH). Nevertheless, regarding the provision aspect, the NHS contracts out and in general, private providers are widely used.

Table 1.1 Healthcare centralisation in different countries

Bangladesh (1996/97)

Revenue collection	General taxation	Donors	Out-of-pocket		Other
Pooling	Ministry of health	Other governmental	No pooling		
Purchasing			Individual purchasing		
Provision	Ministry of health		Private providers		

Chile (1991–1997)

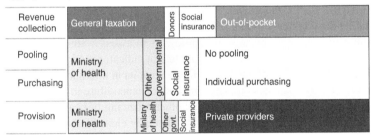

Revenue collection	General taxation	Social insurance	Out-of-pocket
Pooling	Public health insurance fund (FONASA)	Private insurance (ISAPREs)	No pooling
Purchasing			Individual purchasing
Provision	Other governmental	National health service	Private providers

Egypt (1994/95)

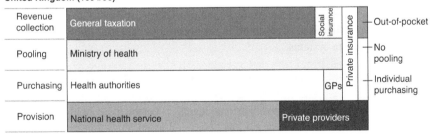

Revenue collection	General taxation	Donors	Social insurance	Out-of-pocket
Pooling	Ministry of health	Other governmental	Social insurance	No pooling
Purchasing				Individual purchasing
Provision	Ministry of health	Ministry of health / Other govt. / Social insurance		Private providers

United Kingdom (1994/95)

Revenue collection	General taxation	Social insurance	Private insurance	Out-of-pocket
Pooling	Ministry of health			No pooling
Purchasing	Health authorities	GPs		Individual purchasing
Provision	National health service	Private providers		

Note: Widths are proportional to estimated flows of funds

Source: National health accounts estimates

Reprinted with permissions from *World Health Report 2000* (WHO 2000, p. 102)

The differences between healthcare systems as depicted in Table 1.1 are striking. Bangladesh and Egypt have an equal mix of public and private in every respect. There are also differences in the types of public and private funding, such as the use of social insurance instead of general taxation. It is also interesting to note that social insurance not only contributes to financing healthcare, but it also plays an important role in pooling and purchasing operations.

Another important observation is that the proportion between public and private is similar for all the factors. Where there is a prevalence of public funding, the other three factors – pooling, purchasing and provision – are also likely to be administered publicly. Of course, as we just argued, this mix might differ due to healthcare dimensions.

A final comment regards the differences even within factors. Social insurance varies significantly from country to country. Some countries may have a system completely administered by the government, while in others a pluralistic social insurance system with competitive forces may exist.[2] However, this can alter the classification of a system from public to societal or mixed.[3] A major methodological difficulty is how to weigh the criteria/factors in order to fit a classification. For example, when it comes to funding: Which is the right financing classification for Egypt or Bangladesh? One way to approach such a question with more accuracy is to concentrate on qualitative rather than quantitative analysis. In other words, classification is, to an extent, a matter of interpretation.

However, very informative quantitative data sources exist that help us to classify healthcare systems with some degree of accuracy. The OECD and World Bank provide detailed data on many health indicators. Some of them are revealing and crucial in the present context because they allow us to assess systems based on preference utilitarian principles. One important health indicator used for the ranking of healthcare systems is healthcare spending per capita in international dollars (Intl$). A similar type of dataset comprises healthcare expenditure in relation (%) to GDP, out of pocket health expenditure, and other financing of healthcare indicators. Figure 1.1 below is an expansion of the financing element. As we can see from Figure 1.1, in the OECD average (in red) approximately more than one third is funded by government taxation, similarly one third by social security, and only approximately one quarter is left to private financing.

Another seminal field of research in healthcare has focussed on the centralisation of healthcare systems.

> Decentralisation can be defined in general terms as the transfer of authority, or dispersal of power, in public planning, management and decision making from the national level to subnational levels . . . On the philosophical and ideological level, decentralisation has been seen as an important political ideal, providing the means for community participation and local self-reliance, and ensuring the accountability of government officials to the population. On a pragmatic level, decentralisation has been seen as a way of overcoming institutional, physical and administrative constraints on development.
>
> (Mills et al. 1990, pp. 12–13)

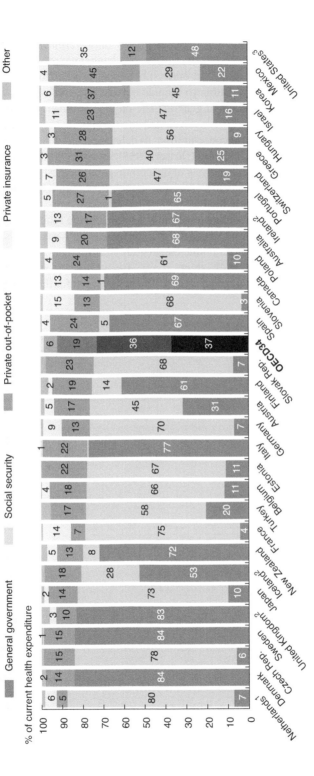

Figure 1.1 Financing of healthcare systems. Expenditure on health by type of financing, 2013 (or nearest year).

Source: OECD (2015)

Decentralisation in this manner focusses mainly on government functions. It enhances the choice of citizens and strengthens the democratic processes by more direct decision-making at local and other subnational levels. However, decentralisation can be expanded further to include outsourcing and more active participation by the private sector in general. The public administration approach, advocated by Mills et al. (1990), has developed into a well-known typology of four forms of decentralisation: i) deconcentration, ii) delegation, iii) devolution, and iv) privatisation, applying to healthcare (Bossert 1998). Bossert (1998), in reviewing the major frameworks for the analysis of decentralisation, suggests an innovative framework based on what he calls 'decision space', the scope which the central authority allows for making effective choices. He provides various functions and activities (Table 1.2). In accordance with this framework, the functions of different healthcare systems can be assessed on a preference utilitarian basis, which facilitates the analysis of the economic calculation problem.

Arguably, as indicated in Mills' quote above, decentralisation at the pragmatic level can increase development and wealth. The main reason for that is associated

Table 1.2 Healthcare system functions and choices

Functions	Range of choice		
	narrow	moderate	wide
Finance			
Sources of revenue	→	→	→
Allocation of expenditures	→	→	→
Income from fees and contracts	→	→	→
Service organisation			
Hospital autonomy	→	→	→
Insurance plans	→	→	→
Payment mechanisms	→	→	→
Contracts with private providers	→	→	→
Required programs/norms	→	→	→
Human resources			
Salaries	→	→	→
Contracts	→	→	→
Civil service	→	→	→
Access rules			
Targeting	→	→	→
Governance rules			
Facility boards	→	→	→
Health offices	→	→	→
Community participation	→	→	→

Source: Bossert, *Analyzing the decentralization of health systems in developing countries: decision space, innovation and performance*. Soc. Sci. Med. Vol. 47, No. 10, Elsevier Science (1998).

with the economic calculation problem: decentralisation can assist in the more efficient allocation of economic resources and at the same time reduce bureaucratic transaction costs. Mills et al. (1990) recognise that privatisation is an effective solution: voluntary agencies and private practitioners are capable of attaining resources that the government cannot obtain and of providing more efficiently some services such as curative medicine. However, they examine many case studies of decentralisation across various countries, and they conclude that in practice many variants are possible (Mills et al. 2009).

Another approach for assessing the efficiency of public and private healthcare systems is to directly compare them. However, comparisons are based upon a plethora of healthcare system evaluation categories and subcategories. The variety of performance criteria makes such comparisons complicated; often they do not have common indicators, or they present other methodological limitations. One such important limitation is again the degree to which a healthcare system can be characterised as private or public if there are government regulation, competitive forces etc.

Basu et al. (2012) reviewed the literature on the long-standing and polarising debate on global health with a view to the role and performance of public and private healthcare services. They systematically evaluated more than a hundred studies published from 1980 to 2011 in low- and middle-income countries. They found that in general, there is no support for the claim that the private sector is more efficient, accountable, or medically effective than the public sector, though the latter appears to lack timeliness and hospitality towards patients (Basu et al. 2012). However, it should be noted that private healthcare systems present at least some advantages over public systems. Further research will be required in this direction.

To conclude this section, the world's healthcare systems present many differences from each other. After WWII the two poles, the U.S. and the U.S.S.R., defined different economic, political and healthcare systems. On the one hand, the U.S.S.R. was the closest approximation of socialism, and on the other hand the U.S.A. was the role model of private enterprise and capitalism. Historical events resulted in the introduction of the NHS in the U.K., which subsequently influenced many healthcare systems in the commonwealth and worldwide. The NHS strengthened the influence of the state and the centralisation of healthcare. Similar trends occurred in the U.S. with Medicare and Medicaid. The expansion of both programmes extended the influence of the state and central authority also in the U.S. However, in the U.S. there is a higher level of participation by the private sector. Continental Europe and Scandinavia had a strong tradition of socialism and social democracy. In that sense, all major systems can be regarded as mixed systems: some have a more centralised authority, and others are more decentralised and private.

We have presented some types of classification that could help us to better understand the multiple dimensions and complications associated with the debate on socialism and private exchange markets. It is not an easy task to assess healthcare systems from both the theoretical and practical perspective. However, based on the main criteria used in many related studies, financing and provision of healthcare seems to be dominated by the public sector. Of course, in most cases, healthcare systems feature a mix of elements with socialist characteristics and decentralised initiatives and markets. In general, decentralised healthcare systems provide significantly more choice to individuals than centralised systems. It may also be argued that decentralised systems perform better, especially if we compare the U.S. with the former U.S.S.R. However, since most of modern healthcare systems present a mix of elements, it is harder to assess them in utilitarian terms. Such an assessment would require much more technical research and analysis of the relevant literature, which is beyond the scope of this chapter.

3. Discussion and conclusions

The economic calculation debate sought to prove in theory that decentralised markets are more efficient than socialism. The collapse of the U.S.S.R. provided one historical example frequently interpreted as proving the failure of socialism. However, socialism can be rarely found in its pure form. Social democracy, a middle ground between the socialist and capitalist ends of the political and economic spectrum, often prevailed and can be found in countries such as Denmark or Norway (Nordic model).

Healthcare systems have historically evolved and been shaped by political administrations. The healthcare system classifications have shown that healthcare tends to be closer to socialism rather than capitalism, mainly due to state ownership and central administration. However, in most cases, systems remain mixed. Market functions are embedded in state-run systems at different levels of funding, insurance, provision, and regulation. This is reminiscent of Lange's search for a model of market socialism that can be functional. Nevertheless, in a considerable number of countries adhering to social democracy, healthcare systems rather seem to correspond to socialism. In many of these countries centralisation in administration, regulation, financing, purchasing, and provision in healthcare may be considered very high. Therefore, they are arguably even closer to socialism than the competitive model proposed by Lange and, of course, even more distant from both Mises and Hayek than one might assume.

From a classical-utilitarian standpoint it is crucial to identify the inefficient parts of healthcare systems and how they reduce health and wealth. However, increasing attention should be paid to measuring levels of competition. Competitive forces exist in some healthcare markets, but it is essential to assess how this falls short of perfect competition. This concern features in Lange's model but more so in the Mises-Hayek critique. Competition is regarded as crucial, since Pareto and the laws of welfare economics suggest that without perfect competition we cannot attain the maximisation of either wealth or health.

Competition can be significantly encouraged by the participation of a larger number of organisations. For example, the great contribution of philanthropic organisations in providing healthcare services should not be overlooked. Healthcare decentralisation and competition can be facilitated by the participation of diverse organisations (i.e. profit, not-for profit, government, religious, other phil-anthropic, etc.). A pluralism of organisations would not only encourage competi-tion and therefore economic efficiency, but it would also facilitate innovation in healthcare and better services and practices.

The main question resulting from this analysis is: How do we attain optimum wealth and consequently health in healthcare systems? How can these systems be efficient and hence increase affordability? It seems that decentralised health-care can provide the best solution to reaching this goal. The opportunity cost of adopting another form of inefficient socialist, or even a mixed model, can be substantial.

It is a frequent misconception that decentralised and market systems would not allow for government initiatives. Friedrich von Hayek (1945) in his *tour de force*, *The Road to Serfdom*, argued for the existence of a state safety net:

> There is no reason why in a society which has reached the general level of wealth which ours has attained, the first kind of security [the security which can be provided for all outside of and supplementary to the market system] should not be guaranteed to all without endangering freedom. There are diffi-cult questions about the precise standard which should thus be assured . . . Nor is there any reason why the state should not assist the individual in providing for these common hazards of life against which, because of the uncertainty, few individuals can make adequate provisions.
>
> (p. 124–125)

Pluralism in healthcare organisation can also strengthen the safety net. Non-profit charitable organisations such as the St. Jude Children's Research Hospital in Mem-phis, Tennessee, can make a major contribution to providing healthcare. Other notable charitable organisations include the Red Cross, Doctors without Borders, and the Task Force for Global Heath. Particularly in Africa, religious organisations account for a large part of healthcare.

Economic considerations and discussions should be part of every healthcare system reform. Whilst healthcare systems may be economically optimised, there is space for a political discussion on how to distribute resources and safeguard vulnerable individuals. But such a political discussion should not supersede or preclude the discussion about what is economically viable and affordable. Decen-tralisation and competition of healthcare systems should be an essential part of such a discussion because healthcare flourishes best in a decentralised healthcare system, providing the maximum health and choice for citizens.

Notes

1 However, other methods like cost-effectiveness, while using monetary values for costs, employ other metrics for effectiveness measurement.
2 'Social security organisation (single or multiple, competing or not), mostly relying on salary-related contributions, owning provider networks or purchasing from exter-nal providers, and serving mostly their own members (usually formal sector workers)'

(WHO 2000). This is a form of organisation in healthcare that can have very different forms, and more detail is needed in order to appropriately assess and categorise.

3 As suggested by Wendt et al. (2009).

References

Bambra, C. (2005). Health Status and the Worlds of Welfare. *Social Policy and Society*, Vol. 5, No. 1, pp. 53–62.

Basu, S. et al. (2012). Comparative Performance of Private and Public Healthcare Systems in Low- and Middle-Income Countries: A Systematic Review. *PLoS Med*, Vol. 9, No. 6, pp. 1–14.

Bentham, J. (1789). *An Introduction to the Principles of Morals and Legislation*. Oxford: Clarendon Press.

Blank, R. H. and Burau, V. (2004). *Comparative Health Policy*. London: Palgrave.

Boettke, P. (1998). Economic Calculation: The Austrian Contribution to Political Economy. *Advances in Austrian Economics*, Vol. 5, pp. 131–158.

Bossert, T. (1998). Analyzing the Decentralization of Health Systems in Developing Countries: Decision Space, Innovation and Performance. *Social Science & Medicine*, Vol. 47, No. 10, pp. 1513–1527.

Brutzkus, B. D. (1921–22). Problemy narodnogo khozyaistva pri sotsialisticheskom stroe. *Ekonomist (Russkoe tekhnicheskoe obshchestvo)*, (Moscow 1921–22), No. 1, pp. 48–65, No. 2, pp. 163–183, No. 3, p. 5.

Burau, V. and Blank, R. H. (2006). Comparing Health Policy: An Assessment of Typologies of Health Systems. *Journal of Comparative Policy Analysis*, Vol. 8, No. 1, pp. 63–76.

Esping-Andersen, G. (1990). *The Three Worlds of Welfare Capitalism*. Cambridge: Polity Press.

Field, M. G. (1973). The Concept of the 'Health System' at the Macrosociological Level. *Social Science and Medicine*, Vol. 7, pp. 763–785.

Friedenberg, D. S. (1987). Soviet Health System. *Western Journal of Medicine*, Vol. 147, No. 2, pp. 214–217.

Giaimo, S. and Manow, P. (1999). Adapting the Welfare State: The Case of Health Care Reform in Britain, Germany, and the United States. *Comparative Political Studies*, Vol. 32, No. 8, pp. 967–1000.

Hayek, F. A. (ed.). (1935). *Collectivist Economic Planning*. London: Routledge and Sons.

Hayek, F. A. (1940). Socialist Calculation: The Competitive 'Solution'. *Economica, New Series*, Vol. 7, No. 26, pp. 125–149.

Hayek, F. A. (1945). The Use of Knowledge in Society. *The American Economic Review*, Vol. 35, No. 4, pp. 519–530.

Lange, O. (1936). On the Economic Theory of Socialism. *Review of Economic Studies*, Vol. 4, pp. 53–71.

Mills, A. et al. (eds.). (1990). *Health System Decentralization: Concepts, Issues and Country Experience*. Geneva: World Health Organisation.

Mises, von L. (1920). *Economic Calculation in the Socialist Commonwealth*. Available at: https://mises.org/library/economic-calculation-socialist-commonwealth/html/c/9 [last accessed 10 August 2017]

Mises, von L. (1940). *Human Action*. Auburn, AL: Mises Institute.

Moran, M. (1999). *Governing the Health Care State: A Comparative Study of the United Kingdom, the United States and Germany*. Manchester: Manchester University Press.

OECD (1987). *Financing and Delivering Health Care: A Comparative Analysis of OECD Countries*. Paris: OECD Publishing.

OECD (2015). Financing of Health Care. In: *Health at a Glance 2015: OECD Indicators*. Paris: OECD Publishing. DOI: http://dx.doi.org/10.1787/health_glance-2015-graph156-en

Olson, M. (1965). *The Logic of Collective Action: Public Goods and the Theory of Groups*. Cambridge, MA: Harvard University Press.

Ostrom, E. (1990). *Governing the Commons: The Evolution of Institutions for Collective Action*. Cambridge: Cambridge University Press.

Rowland, D. and Telyukov, A. V. (1991). Soviet Health Care from Two Perspectives. *Health Affairs*, Vol. 10, No. 3, pp. 71–86.

Weber, M. (1921). *Economy and Society*. Berkeley, CA: University of California Press.

Wendt, K., Frisina, L., and Rothgang, H. (2009). Healthcare System Types: A Conceptual Framework for Comparison. *Social Policy & Administration*, Vol. 43, No. 1, pp. 70–90.

WHO (2000). *The World Health Report 2000*. Geneva: WHO, p. 102, Fig. 5.2 Structure of health system financing and provision in four countries.

2   The corruption of medical morality under advanced capitalism

Miran Epstein

1. Terminology

To prevent ambiguity and confusion, some of the basic terms to be used in the following are defined and explicated at the very outset.

Social consciousness is the collective mental-functional expression of any particular social relations: it reflects and mediates them in some way. A *collective* is any "ensemble of social relations" (Marx, 1969, VI). A collective may appear as a society, community, organisation, group, or individual.

The term *ideology* has received different meanings some of which are loaded and even pejorative (Eagleton, 1991). Here it refers neutrally to the body of ideas that correspond to any particular consciousness.

Moral consciousness (*morality, conscience*) is the kind of consciousness that grasps social relations in moral terms. Historically, it is the collective self-regulating, self-judging, self-enforcing, and self-affirming consciousness of some social compromise. As such, it is necessarily distorted and distorting: it perceives only the *fair* aspects of the compromise and thus grasps the compromise itself as if it were fair, when in fact it never is. Compromises are shaped by power, not fairness.

Ethic (plural *ethics*) is the ideological expression of moral consciousness and the benchmark by which it makes its moral judgments. It consists of *rules* (dos and don'ts) as well as *their moral justifications* (moral values, moral theories and tools, and moral authorities, e.g. God or moral reason). It is expressed in spoken language, religious texts, oaths, codes, declarations, policies, doctrines, and/or laws. It is of, by, and for the pertinent collective, it expresses nothing but common interests, it is binding on all actors equally, and its rules appear as ends in themselves that have been deduced from their moral justifications.[1]

The adjectives *ethical* and *unethical* denote acting in accordance with, or in violation of, any particular ethic and signifying collective approbation and condemnation, respectively. Since the collective uses its ethic as a moral yardstick, it also takes the adjectives to denote *moral* (good) and *immoral* (bad), respectively. However, the statements, 'if it's ethical, then it's moral' and 'if it's unethical then it's immoral', are *non-sequiturs*. Sociological statements entail no necessary metaphysical conclusions.

Medical ethic or *the ethic of medicine* denotes the ethic of any particular medical collective. A *medical collective* covers the entire spectrum of the division of medical labour. Unless otherwise indicated, it is metonymically referred to as *doctors*, their clients being *patients*. The organisation of a medical collective is called *medical system* or *medicine*. These neutral terms replace the loaded term *healthcare system*.

The *ethic of our medicine* – in short, *our ethic* – denotes the hitherto most developed medical ethic, which is an artefact comprising the most developed components of different medical ethics from different countries. Our ethic is expressed in codes, declarations, policies, doctrines and laws. *Our medicine* refers to the medicine to which this ethic corresponds. Our ethic and our medicine are thus abstractions, albeit very real ones.

Capital is the social class that possesses, invests, and amasses *capital*, i.e. money whose purpose is to make more money. *Capitalism* is any kind of Capital-dominated economic-cultural social formation. *Capitalist medicine* is any kind of medicine that is subjected to the logic of Capital whether directly (because it is dependent thereon) or indirectly (because it is impoverished thereby), or both. *Humanist medicine* is a medicine that treats its patient as a human being, and not as labour power, customer, guinea pig, source of biological commodities, or financial liability.

2. The ostensible paradox

> We came here to serve God, and also to get rich.
> (attributed to Bernal Díaz del Castillo)[2]

> All science would be superfluous if the outward appearance and the essence of things directly coincided.
> (Karl Marx)[3]

Our ethical medicine displays what appears to be a perplexing paradox. On the one hand, it vows to put the patient first. On the other hand, it abuses the patient and the doctor too, though not necessarily in each and every case. Moreover, the harm it inflicts on them is much more alarming than the harm inflicted on them by its corrupt sister. Like the latter, it abandons them to the mercy of Capital, a stakeholder for whom benefit and harm to people are both different means to, as well as different consequences of, its inherently exploitative end. Only it does it on a much larger scale, and with a smile. We, patients and doctors, rarely put this perplexity into words, but we often feel it in our bones. To both of us, medicine and its ethic seem to be standing vis-à-vis one another like the face and the vase in the famous shifting blind spot cognitive-optical illusion developed by the Danish psychologist Edgar Rubin more than a hundred years ago: when we look at our medicine through the lens of its sublime ethic we see none of its offensive aspects, but when we turn to these aspects we no longer see any ethic (Rubin, 1915).

Let us take a closer look at this enigma, starting with its ethical arm.

The World Medical Association (WMA) commands that the health of the patient be the physician's "first consideration" (World Medical Association, 2006). It also states that the primary goals of medical research "can never take precedence over the rights and interests of individual research subjects" (World Medical Association, 2013). The same goes for the American Medical Association (AMA). It instructs the physician to "regard responsibility to the patient as paramount" (American Medical Association, 2001). The British General Medical Council (GMC) does so too. "Make the care of the patient your first concern", it insists (General Medical Council, 2013a). The British National Health Service (NHS) goes further, making a systemic commitment: "The NHS aspires to put patients at the heart of everything it does" (NHS Core Principles, 2011).

And by no means are these words empty. Each and every one of the rules of the ethic indeed expresses a tangible patient liberty: patients are normally allowed to decline proposed interventions; they can expect their doctors to protect their privacy from relatives, employers, and the general public; they are entitled to be treated fairly, free from arbitrariness and undue bias; they can rely on oversight bodies to safeguard them from certain risks; they can have their unwanted pregnancies terminated; if the worst comes to the worst, they can even request assistance in suicide or euthanasia. Each of these liberties somehow serves the patients. None of them are fake. They are real, because they feel real. Moreover, while the common intuitive assumption that these liberties and their corresponding ethic are both necessarily and actually emancipatory will be contested in the following, their emancipatory potential cannot be denied.

But once we shift to the practical arm of the ostensible paradox, an offensive picture comes to light. What we see here is the Capital-driven pervasive commercialisation and privatisation of medicine and their disturbing implications: perverted agendas of clinical medicine, biomedical research and the biomedical industry, distortion of medical knowledge, declining access to adequate care, deteriorating quality of care, and widening rich-poor health inequalities. What is striking about these anti-patient and doctor trends is that none of them necessarily involve impropriety. On the contrary, they typically occur with all the checks and balances in place. They usually abide by the ethic piously, and yet they render its emancipatory promise null and void. They reduce each of the liberties it expresses to a cynical shell.

Let there be no mistake: we are not dealing here with capitalist (or any other) corruption. True, many cases of corruption in our medicine (and elsewhere) and certainly the most serious ones carry the fingerprints of Capital, and most of them indeed harm us all (Gøtzsche, 2013; Goldacre, 2012; Angell, 2005; Kassirer, 2005). There is also no doubt that capitalist corruption can render the ethic incapable of delivering on its promises. Equally undeniable is the fact that Capital often buys (ethically) or bribes (unethically) the Legislature, the Executive, and the Judiciary, turning them into its private handmaidens who would not only streamline its ethical ventures but also go easy on its improprieties, making the punishment a financial risk possibly worth taking. That Capital tolerates and indeed profits from a moderate rate of corruption of any kind is indisputable too (Reiner, 2006). But corruption attests to nothing but the intensity of human drives. As a matter of fact, it is marginal in both medicine and capitalism and is certainly immanent in neither. Moreover, a totally ethicless capitalist medicine is inconceivable, whereas a perfectly ethical capitalist medicine is easily conceivable, and yet precisely herein lies the mystery we are dealing with.

Take, for example, the British medical system, which many countries rightly regard with envy. Its central ethical text, *Good Medical Practice*, presupposes and conveys the message that the compliant system is *good*, both for its patients and for its staff (General Medical Council, 2013b). No doubt, when looked at from the vantage point of this text, the system seems perfectly harmonious. But, lo and behold, it, its patients and staff are subjected to an unprecedentedly severe capitalist onslaught, *an onslaught that in no way interferes with Good Medical Practice, and yet undermines the very possibility of good medical practice* (see, for example, Hiam et al., 2017). Isn't that a paradox?

3. Mainstream denials and explanations

To dispute the premises of the ostensible paradox and deny its very existence one may simply assert that the ethic is indeed patient-centred. This position is implicit in the way we perceive the ethic and teach it. Alternatively, one may contend that our medicine is, as a matter of fact, patient-centred. After all, a truly patient-centred ethic implies a truly patient-centred medicine, and vice versa. This position is typical of patients and doctors who draw general conclusions from their private, genuinely or just reputedly, positive experience. A thousand times different, it is also typical of barefaced government officials and medical managers who reaffirm the system's 'commitment to excellent care' whenever they introduce new cuts and other anti-patient and -doctor measures. Either way, there is no paradox. Our ethical medicine is a coherent idyll.

Indeed, the ostensible paradox has rarely been identified as such, and explicit attempts to explain it away are hard to come by. Nevertheless, the bioethical discourse implies two possible explanations.

One explanation attributes the ostensible paradox to misperception of the interface between two different public wills. First, the public wants to put Capital first. Is this not what it voted for? Second, it wants doctors to put the patient first. An ostensible paradox appears only to those who wrongly think that these wills have a common history or that they are actually contradictory. In truth, so it is suggested, they are historically independent from each other; they coexist adventitiously. And, as each pertains to a different object, they are also mutually inclusive. Bioethicists who advance this sort of explanation regard the status quo as an outcome of democratic, and hence irreproachable, choices. To doctors who are unhappy with it they say, 'express your concerns at the ballot box'.

The second explanation attributes the ostensible paradox to the false assumption that the ethic is foolproof. Proponents of this explanation posit that medicine is insufficiently patient-centred, because its ethic, contrary to its appearance, is lax. Many of them are convinced that the problems of our medicine boil down to regulatory cracks and loopholes that can fortunately be fixed.

> The current regulations – for companies, doctors and researchers – create perverse incentives; and we'll have better luck fixing those broken systems than we will ever have trying to rid the world of avarice.
>
> (Goldacre, 2012, p. 11)

Others feel that the ethic is broken beyond repair. Disillusioned with focal regulatory antidotes, some blame it for failing to restrain Capital, while others accuse it of accommodating to its whims. Both ask us to take one step back. To save our medicine, they say, we must restore its traditional ethic.

> Profits threaten to preempt the personal, the professional, and more fundamentally still, the ethical dimension of the patient-physician relationship . . . . [The] main challenge facing medicine [is] that of ensuring that free-market medicine remains moral medicine and that medical ethics rises to the challenge of preserving medicine's moral mandate within the context of managed care.
>
> (Baker et al., 1999)

> Fidelity to the moral center of medicine is the only antidote to the moral malaise that afflicts our profession today. We do not need a "new" ethic of accommodation to economics, commerce, or the idolatry of the marketplace. Even less do our patients need such an ethic.
>
> (Pellegrino, 1999)

> The bioethics that might have been would not have thought to displace the older ethic of medicine but instead to expand upon its general moral vision . . . . Had bioethicists done that they might have created a moral space within which the balance between economic imperatives and human necessities could even be considered.
>
> (Koch, 2012; see also Koch, 2014)

Notwithstanding their differences, these explanations presuppose that the relations between the ethic and Capital are accidentally symbiotic. Commendably or condemnably, they maintain *elective affinity* (*Wahlverwandtschaft*).[4] The ethic is indeed compatible with, and perhaps even conducive to, capitalist interests, but only by sheer historical coincidence.

This view is becoming increasingly common (Kutcher, 2009; Imber, 2008; Rothman, 2003; Bosk, 2002; Evans, 2001; Stevens, 2000; Rosenberg, 1999; Bosk, 1999; Imber, 1998; Guillemin, 1998; Kleinman, 1995; Callahan, 1993). It entertains the possibility of a coherent ethical medicine. It also presupposes that a capitalist medicine can, in principle, have a patient-centred ethic. On both counts, it gets it wrong.

4. A social theory of moral consciousness

All forms of social consciousness arise from, echo, and mediate material aspects of social life. In other words, they are their historical psychological-functional expressions. Moral consciousness is no exception.

> [Men], developing their material production and their material intercourse, alter, along with this their real existence, their thinking and the products of their thinking. Life is not determined by consciousness, but consciousness by life.
>
> (Marx, 1932)

To understand any particular moral consciousness means to uncover its social roots. For that, one needs a general theory of moral consciousness and a deductive method. The theory must be historical (explanatory), and not philosophical (justificatory). It does not concern itself with the truth value of moral consciousness.[5] Nor does it make any moral assumptions or draw any moral conclusions.

The theory maintains that moral consciousness is the collective mental-regulatory expression of some compromise. To explain this point, let us note that every compromise implies the following conditions:

(1) The relations among the actors rest on some irreconcilable conflicts and therefore involve power.
(2) In addition to, and possibly also subject to, their power relations, the actors somehow depend on each other and therefore have some common ground.
(3) The power gap seems to them neither too wide nor too narrow.

Clearly, these conditions entail some compromise and determine its particular nature. Changes in them may thus result in a new compromise, violent oppression, war, or total harmony. Anyway, like any other aspect of social life, compromises have two tiers.

The primary tier is *material*. It involves both material concessions on behalf of, as well as material achievements for, each of the actors. It is expressed in material relations and material institutions. Its concrete nature – the scope of the consensus – is shaped by the material interests involved and their relative power. This vector equation creates the compromise in its own image and thereby reinforces itself. By replacing its originally violent glue with the more reliable adhesive of consensus, it turns itself into *cooperative power relations* (Stewart, 2001).

The secondary tier of the compromise is *psychological*. It consists of the mental expressions of the material tier, namely the ways in which the collective perceives it and the ideology that corresponds to these perceptions. When fully developed, the psychological tier of a compromise typically consists of different forms of collective consciousness, e.g. descriptive, explanatory, etc. However, moral consciousness is its quintessential feature. All other forms may also develop under circumstances that involve no compromise. Moral consciousness cannot. Moreover, the moral consciousness of a material compromise presides over its other mental expressions.[6]

The collective as such can only see the consensual aspects of the compromise. The non-consensual aspects cannot be grasped collectively. The development of this tubular vision and peripheral blindness does not require deception. Nor does it involve suppression, denial, or self-delusion.

The process starts with the parties seeing the full picture. What holds the compromise together is fear of the alternatives, with fear being a poor stabiliser. If the compromise survives long enough, the parties will come to perceive it as rational. Rationality is a poor stabiliser too.[7] Given more time, though, the price for acting rationally (and thus also inconsistently) will turn out to be too heavy to pay. To protect themselves, the parties increasingly act automatically. At this stage, the order and its distorted-distorting consciousness are produced and reproduced increasingly through *hegemony* and *interpellation*.[8] Force takes the back seat, ready to be unleashed if the circumstances require. Each party is still aware of its own gains and losses, but they can no longer see the historical connection between them. The losses divide them, but the benefits unite them. When they look at the benefits they see common interests; they see them collectively. But the collective vantage point also makes them see things upside down: as if the order tallied with their collective will, as if it were harmonious, and as if it were an end in itself. By breeding this psychological inversion, the order actually reinforces and perpetuates itself.[9]

Of course, the corresponding ideology must mirror this inverted perception accurately. For example, the rules of the compromise are bound to focus on its sanguine side only, i.e. the common interests on which it rests. Understandably, they are also destined to side with the most disenfranchised party and play up its miserable achievements.[10] In any case, the rules are compelled to treat the irreconcilable differences, i.e. the non-negotiable matters, with silence. And though they may possibly allude to certain conflicts, they cannot relate to the power relations, the power balance, any demands – successful or failed – the parties cannot agree upon, how the material compromise allocates benefits and burdens, its history, and even its very fact. No wonder the rules acquire a *moral form*, appearing as if they were ends in themselves, deduced from some moral values, and handed over by some supreme moral authority. No wonder we fetishise them, treat them as if they created us in their own image, when in fact it is the other way around. No wonder they merely 'manage' the compromise, and never ever confront it.

It turns out, then, that the collective consciousness of any material compromise, including moral consciousness, is in fact a corresponding psychological compromise negotiated by the same vector equation. This consciousness is 'necessarily false', to use the classic Marxian adjective pertaining to any consciousness that is distorted by power relations and therefore necessarily distorts them and thereby preserves them.

5. The power of the theory

The theory presented above explains in general why morality appears or not; how it acquires its moral form; why it may change, disappear, or reappear; why different social relations may give rise to similar or different moralities and ethics; why similar relations may give rise to different or similar moralities and ethics; and why certain relations can give rise to different moralities and ethics, but not to any morality and ethic. The theory also explains why ethical relations necessarily give rise to an ostensible paradox – a disparity between their harmonious form and their disharmonious content. It explains why this disparity is immanent in all ethical relations, and why it is a universal feature thereof. Further, the theory explains why, in quiet times, the prevailing ethical discourse is bound to be predominantly philosophical-justificatory and not historical-explanatory, and why the mainstream historiography of the ethic would be inclined to produce distorted explanations. The theory can even explain its own currently poor social status and describe, in general, the conditions that could make it increasingly acceptable.

As stated above, the theory entails no necessary philosophical implications. However, it entails several far-reaching conclusions of theoretical importance.

It explains why all ethics necessarily seem humanist. However, it concludes that, since an ethic is an expression of a certain compromise, it can only be as humanist as the latter.

Let there be no misunderstanding. The fact that all ethics express, distort, and sanction power relations does not mean that every ethic is necessarily misanthropic. Whether it is misanthropic or humanist depends on the nature of the power relations it affirms. If it affirms misanthropic power relations, namely relations wherein particularistic interests prevail over universal interests, then it is misanthropic. If it affirms humanist power relations, i.e. relations wherein universal interests prevail over particularistic interests or even over other universal interests, then it is humanist.

Further, since humanist and misanthropic compromises can equally give rise to a seemingly sublime ethic, and since every ethic can possibly turn out to be playing a misanthropic role, the theory warns us to never take any ethic at face value and to approach all ethics at all times with extreme caution.[11]

Equally, the theory instructs us to never judge any social order by its ethic, but rather to judge the ethic by the order it sanctions. Since every ethic is an alluring distorted-distorting manifestation of some compromise, it can only be understood in its light. What an ethic expresses (the fairness of the playing) can thus make sense only in the light of what it treats with silence (the unfairness of the game). Considered in the abstract, it is as meaningless as 'a grin without a cat' (Carroll, 1979). Considering it in the abstract may be dangerous.

Following from that, the theory teaches us that a critique of social relations must be immanent: it must rest on the heuristic assumption that they are perfectly ethical, even if this is not always the case. It is not a big deal to criticise the master for stealing from his slaves. The real challenge is to criticise him for exploiting them.

The theory also has something to say to the moral philosopher and the applied ethicist. The philosophical question is, in the final analysis, a historical question.[12] This does not necessarily render philosophy redundant. However, it entails that it can be truly critical only if it is informed by its own social role, i.e. the role it plays in the context of its reception.

The theory addresses activists too. First, it reveals to us that, since the ethic is merely an expression of some context, a meaningful change of the ethic or a change of its meaning alone can take place only if the context is ripe. Thus, regardless of how radical an ethical change may seem, it can only be as radical as the contextual change. Second, the theory predicts that, once the context has been exposed, it might make us see the morality and its ethic in a different light. The theory entertains the possibility that, as a result, we may perhaps become critical of them. However, it entails that such a development could not by itself make us abandon them. Indeed, as long as the social circumstances persist, so will their consciousness and its ideology, no matter how critical of them we may be (Marx, 1990, pp. 163–177). Thirdly, and most important, the theory teaches us that the circumstances, and not their consciousness, should be the primary focus of our critical attention and political action. Most specifically, it instructs the humanist to never separate the struggle for a humanist consciousness from the struggle for a humanist society.

> The philosophers have only interpreted the world, in various ways; the point is to change it.
>
> (Marx, 1969, XI)

6. From intuition to method

Since the only thing that distinguishes humanist ethics from misanthropic ones is their contexts, getting the context of an ethic right is of utmost theoretical and practical importance. Yet, since the context always hides behind the cloak of the ethic, it must be determined not by intuition but by some rational method. The theory entails this method.

The method rests on the understanding that, since the ethic is an expression of some compromise, each is likely to leave some fingerprints on the other. A 'forensic' examination of the ethic may thus point to some suspect compromise. Now, if we can show that the latter actually exists in some concrete form, and provide convincing evidence connecting it causally to the ethic, we will be able to confirm the suspicion with high confidence.[13]

The method has two stages, then. The first stage – the inquiry – is analytic-reconstructive, i.e. sociological. If successful, it should culminate in a *historical theory* of the ethic, a theory that regards the ethic tentatively as an expression of the suspect compromise. The second stage – the presentation – must be synthetic-constructive, i.e. historical. It forms the test of the theory, which, however plausible, would otherwise remain speculative. This stage requires us to produce a *history* of the ethic – a historical-causal narrative constructing the ethic from the suspect compromise – using the historical theory generated in the previous stage as a scaffold to be supported by hard evidence. If this goes well, we will be able to corroborate the theory. At this point, the concrete object – the ethical compromise – will reveal itself to us in all clarity.[14]

Four comments about this counterintuitive method: First, in its abstract form, it is in fact the *universal method of science*. Second, its synthetic stage cannot furnish, and must not claim to have furnished, the necessary and sufficient conditions for the phenomenon in question. Thus, contrary to common positivistic conceptions, science must avoid making deterministic claims. It should merely seek to convince us that the phenomenon had a *good chance* of emerging in a reality containing the conditions it points to. Third, science aims to expose the essence behind the appearance. It is not after the truth, nor would it be able to identify the truth even if it exists and it were to stumble upon it. In any case, the social fate of knowledge systems and ideas depends not on their truth value but on the economy of interests whose approval they seek. Finally, notwithstanding the last point, science is neither infallible nor indisputable. Nor should it resist change or even abandonment in the light of improved analysis and/or new information.

7. Whose ethic is it anyway?

The central contention of this chapter – that the ostensibly patient-centred ethic of our medicine is, as a matter of fact, a capitalist ethic, i.e. an ethic of, by, and for a capitalist medicine – is not trivial at all. Needless to say, it can make no sense to those who believe that form (ethic) and content (medicine) are historically independent from each other, or that they are bound to coincide, or that the content develops from the form.

The contention is not trivial, even if one accepts the abstract premise that a capitalist medicine is bound to have some pseudo-patient-centred ethic. Who knows, this may not apply to our medicine after all. That it is strongly affected by Capital and that Capital cares not in the least about the patient and the doctor no one can deny. However, this does not necessarily make our medicine 'capitalist'. Indeed, it contains and is shaped by other actors as well.[15] How are we to proceed, then? What do we need to do in order to support the contention?

The process involves three steps:

(1) showing that the ethic presupposes some Capital-dominated compromise, i.e. some capitalist medicine;
(2) showing that such a compromise indeed exists in reality; and
(3) showing that the ethic actually developed from and along with this compromise.

Now let us be more specific.

Let us note that, while the ethic implies some material concessions on behalf of Capital, it contains not even a single anti-capitalist rule – for example, a rule that outlaws any form of for-profit medicine and profit-making in medicine; indeed, such rules are being constantly proposed but repeatedly rejected. Moreover, the capitalist ventures that are implicit in them actually exist and are harmful to the patient and the doctor.

Let us also note that, while the rules of the ethic invariably offer some benefit to each and every party, they rest on abstract premises, fictitious presumptions, and exceptions that give additional advantage to Capital, again in ways that are often detrimental to the patient and the doctor. Here are some key examples, in brief:

Informed consent presupposes autonomy. However, it does not imply autonomy. Its tests of autonomy are based on fictitious presumptions. Even worse, the conditions for realising these presumptions exist only rarely, primarily owing to the sundry perfectly ethical capitalist ventures that manipulate the values and desires of people, corrupt their knowledge, and distort and/or restrict their options. Let us note that the doctrine reflects contractual relations in which the patient is, or resembles a customer. Let us also note that, though the capitalist market must deem most customers autonomous, it cannot tolerate the idea that only the autonomous ones be allowed to shop. As mentioned in the previous paragraph, it tries hard to render them heteronomous. The doctrine of informed consent fits this twisted bill; by branding choice as free choice, it affirms imposition of responsibility on those who are not and cannot be responsible for their choices. (Epstein, 2006; Epstein, 2016). It should come as no surprise, then, that the shift from the fiduciary ethic of 'best interests' to the contractual ethic of consent coincided in time and place with the transition of medicine from the capitalist sphere of production to the capitalist sphere of exchange, a transition that was driven by Capital in an attempt to increase its share of wealth under historical circumstances that have made this endeavour more difficult in some respects and less so in others. Interestingly, similar transformations have taken place in parallel in other social domains as well, affecting the relationships between parents and children, men and women, white people and others, teachers and students, and more. The medical case is thus but a specific instance of a general historical trend, which, among other things, is turning all ethics into subspecies of a single global ethic: business ethic.

The duty of medical confidentiality suggests a medicine that protects patient privacy in the broadest sense of the word. In practice, however, Capital increasingly treats personal medical information as its private commodity. The fiction of opt-out consent allows it to do this ethically (Hawkes, 2011). Patient privacy is thus reduced to protection from simple gossip.

The ethic of rationing suggests that scarcity is an outcome of the inevitable gap between demand and supply, when in fact it is primarily an artefact of Capital's wealth-redistribution strategy. Moreover, the supreme criterion of the ethic, 'cost-effectiveness' (maximum effectiveness at minimum cost), sounds rational, humanist, and unobjectionable. However, 'effectiveness' is measured neither in life expectancy nor in subjective happiness, but in Quality-Adjusted Life-Years (QALYs), a standard of economic productivity construed as contribution to 'growth', i.e. profit (National Institute for Health and care Excellence, 2013).

While these points are merely suggestive of capital's involvement, it is a fact that the criterion was originally put forward by no one else but the World Bank, as part of its successful global attempt to funnel more wealth from the poor majority to an increasingly small and insatiable minority (The World Bank, 1993).

Our end-of-life ethic appeals to the sublime 'right to die with dignity'. But the message that this right conveys in an economy based on austerity, privatisation, and commercialisation – an economy that scorns the 'right to live with dignity' and regards poor incurable patients as an intolerable financial burden – is very different: buy or die! (Epstein, 2007). It turns out, then, that this ethic is effectively an extension of the ethic of rationing.

The ethic of medical research, drug approval, marketing, and pricing presupposes a mostly profit-driven system. Ridden with abstractions, legal fictions, exceptions and contradictions, it works primarily for Capital often to the detriment of the human guinea pig and the patient.

For example, notwithstanding the risk of bias (and corruption), the ethic allows the medical party to have financial conflicts of interest. It allows subject recruitment through financial incentives. It has no problem with researchers seeking consent from a ludicrous fiction called 'professional legal representative' or even waiving consent altogether, whenever obtaining it is "impossible or impracticable" or "the research cannot be delayed" (World Medical Association, 2013). Under certain conditions, the ethic tolerates any risk to the human guinea pig, however high it may be, even in the absence of any expected benefit. It is silent about seeding trials – that is, marketing exercises concealed as scientific research – and equally about medicalisation and "me too" drugs. It says nothing about the adequacy of selection criteria, outcome measures, statistical significance, and other variables often used to manipulate evidence. It is effectively willing to establish efficacy of a drug merely on the basis of its performance against placebo. It requires 'substantial evidence of efficacy', rather than 'evidence of substantial efficacy'. The next development in the ethic – abandoning the safety hurdle – is pending:

> When you have a drug, you can actually get it approved if it works, instead of waiting for many, many years . . . . We're going to be cutting regulations at a level that nobody's ever seen before, and we're going to have tremendous protection for the people.
>
> (Thomas, 2017, quoting U.S. President Donald Trump)

The ethic of commercial conflicts of interest presupposes a medicine embarrassed by the fact that its dependence on private money is greater than its dependence on the patient. The ethic of such a medicine must not ask the affected doctors to recuse themselves, but merely to disclose their conflicts. The idea that disclosure can protect the patient from harmful commercial interests is ludicrous, as it rests on the fictitious presumptions that (1) the doctor has identified all the potential conflicts, (2) the patient can distinguish between potential and actual conflicts, and (3) the patient can tell, in case of actual conflict, whose interest prevails. The only thing disclosure can do is foster trust in the untrustworthy.

The ethic of organ transplantation speaks primarily on behalf of the suffering patient on the waiting list. However, it presupposes a medicine whose interests are primarily economic: saving on haemodialysis and, in certain systems, profiting from transplantation. So keen is it to get its hand on replacement organs, that it is even willing to make do with inferior ones and to embrace the ethical fictions of altruism and opt-out consent. For quite some time now, it has been entertaining the idea of extending the logic and the ethic of the commodity market to body parts.

The ethic of reproduction suggests a liberated woman. But when we reproduce the woman from the list of her acknowledged rights, we end up with a buyer or a seller, and if neither, then a financial burden – in short, *homo capitalismus*, not a free human being.

The ethic of deinstitutionalisation – the policy of treating physically and mentally disabled people in the community rather than in a public institution – seems a humanitarian measure designed to enable these people to lead the life they much prefer. But the compliant reality is about spending cuts and *de facto* privatisation.

The ethic of 'outsourcing' and 'decentralisation' suggests improved service combined with increased doctor and patient autonomy. The compliant practice, however, indicates government parsimony, *de facto* privatisation, the financialisation of clinical reason, worsening service, and autonomy that expands systematically in relation to money-saving and money-making choices only.

These points strongly suggest a new historical theory of the ethic. The theory incorporates many of the factors that have been mentioned in the mainstream historiography of the ethic. However, it posits that the ethic has been shaped *also and predominantly* by Capital, a player whose role in its history has so far been largely belittled if not ignored altogether.

8. Conclusions

Using a powerful theory of morality and guided by the universal method of science, this chapter has suggested that Capital's greatest harm to patients and doctors occurs under the radar and auspices of an ethic that vows to put us at the centre, and that is not accidental. Nor is it through any fault of the ethic. Our medical ethic is in fact a historical ideological-functional expression of, by, and for a capitalist medicine. Such a medicine cannot have a patient-centred ethic, but it must appear as if it were patient-centred and give rise to an ethic that would affirm this false appearance.

In other words, our capitalist medicine necessarily generates *a gap between how its ethic depicts it and what it really is*. The ethic portrays it as an idyllic win-win game because the collective eye can only see the harmony. But precisely because of that, the ethic does not and cannot give us the full picture. It necessarily conceals from us the fact that the harmony is embedded in and subjected to a rigged zero-sum capitalist master game. In doing so, the ethic effectively reinforces and perpetuates this game.

This gap reduces the ethic to an apologia for a medicine that is in fact a far cry from the one we can have and deserve to have. It turns the ethic, which is in itself meaningless, into a collective ideological narcotic that relieves some of the pain that the callous capitalist medicine inflicts upon us, while making us too inebriated to diagnose the disease correctly, let alone to treat it rationally. It effectively helps Capital transform the decent doctor into its unwitting subcontractor and the patient into either a gullible golden egg-laying goose or an acquiescing financial liability. To sum up, it enables the wolf and the sheep to 'sit around the campfire, hold hands and sing Kumbaya' only to make it easier for the former to prey on the latter (Weiss 2006).

However sublime our medical ethic may seem, it cannot be the remedy for our ailing medicine, as it is nothing but a pathological symptom thereof. Moreover, being sick, our medicine cannot have a healthy ethic, and no ethic, old or new, could by itself heal it. The idea that our medicine can be fixed merely by regulatory means is absurd. It presupposes wrongly that a capitalist medicine can, in principle, have a humanist ethic. No, it cannot: "Ye cannot serve God and mammon" (Matthew 6:24). If you wish to have humanist ethic, get yourselves a humanist medicine!

Notes

1 Rules that are not collective are not ethic.
2 Iglesia (1943); Shem (1978).
3 Marx (1967).
4 The expression had first been coined by Johann Wolfgang von Goethe and later adopted by Max Weber. It denotes what they arguably regarded as the tendency of some phenomena that are historically independent of one another to gravitate towards each other (Swedberg, 2005; Weber, 2011).
5 Social theories of religion or atheism are not concerned with the ontological question because neither depends on whether God exists or not.
6 Astronomical conceptions are descriptive-explanatory, not normative-prescriptive. However, in certain times and places holding to the 'wrong' conception was deemed immoral and could cost one dearly.
7 If we regarded murder as unacceptable for rational reasons only, then we would murder each other whenever we thought this was a rational thing to do.
8 Where the survival of the subordinate actors depends on the success of the ruling actor, then even if his success necessarily comes at their expense, they are likely (1) to see no alternative to the status quo, (2) to perceive his particularistic interests as if they were in tune with the common good, and (3) to regard his material dominance as if it were the product of their choice. *Hegemony* denotes this form of material-psychological command (Gramsci, 1971). *Interpellation* is the mode of dissemination of hegemony. It is the social process whereby relations, roles, and ideas are offered to us in such a way that we are encouraged to accept them. Eliciting our consent by means of invisible coercion, it results in the distorted perception that these relations and ideas are authentically ours (Althusser, 2001).
9 The well-known economic power relations in our society necessarily seem to us as if they were products of our democratic choice, when in fact it is the other way around.
10 The ethic of animal experimentation puts animal lovers and rights activists first. It also speaks highly of the 'wellbeing' of the animals, as well as of the 'humane' methods of killing them when they are rendered useless.
11 Some of the worst atrocities in the history of mankind took place under the auspices of some ethic – for example, slavery and its Judeo-Christian ethic, capitalism and its market and business ethics, war and its military ethic, capital punishment and its execution ethic, etc.
12 Whether or not God exists, the question can only arise in a world that needs Him. Asking it in abstraction from that world uncritically serves to reinforce it.

13   The forensic analogy alludes to Locard's Exchange Principle (The Forensic Library).
14   For Marx's depiction of the method see Marx (1990, p. 102, pp. 493–494).
15   A medicine shaped by one actor only would necessarily be ethicless.

References

Althusser, L. (2001 [1971]). Ideology and ideological state apparatuses. In L. Althusser, *Lenin and Philosophy and Other Essays*. New York: Monthly Review Press, pp. 85–126.
American Medical Association (2001). *Principles of Medical Ethics*, VIII. www.ama-assn.org/sites/default/files/media-browser/principles-of-medical-ethics.pdf
Angell, M. (2005). *The Truth about the Drug Companies: How They Deceive Us and What to Do about It*. New York: Random House.
Baker, R., Caplan, A., Emanuel, L. and Latham, S., eds. (1999). *The American Medical Ethics Revolution: How the AMA Code of Ethics Has Transformed Physicians' Relationships to Patients, Professionals, and Society*. Baltimore: The Johns Hopkins University Press, pp. xxxv–xxxvi.
Bosk, C. (1999). Professional ethicist available: Logical, secular, friendly. *Daedalus*, 128(4), pp. 47–67.
Bosk, C. (2002). Now that we have the data, what was the question? *American Journal of Bioethics*, 2(4), pp. 21–23.
Callahan, D. (1993). Why America accepted bioethics. *Hastings Center Report*, 23(6), pp. 8–9.
Carroll, L. (1979 [1865]). *Alice's Adventures in Wonderland and through the Looking Glass*. Maidenhead: Purnell, p. 58.
Eagleton, T. (1991). *An Introduction to Ideology*. London: Verso.
Epstein, M. (2006). Why effective consent presupposes autonomous authorization: A counter-orthodox argument. *Journal of Medical Ethics*, 32, pp. 342–345.
Epstein, M. (2007). Legitimizing the shameful: End-of-life ethics and the political economy of death. *Bioethics*, 21(1), pp. 23–31.
Epstein, M. (2016). Idealist-atomist autonomy and the commercialization of biomedicine. *American Journal of Bioethics*, 16(2), pp. 65–67.
Evans, J. (2001). *Playing God? Human Genetic Engineering and the Rationalization of Public Bioethical Debate*. Chicago: The University of Chicago Press.
The Forensic Library. *Edmond Locard*. http://aboutforensics.co.uk/edmond-locard/
General Medical Council (2013a). *Good Medical Practice*. Duties of a doctor. www.gmc-uk.org/guidance/good_medical_practice/duties_of_a_doctor.asp
General Medical Council (2013b). *Good Medical Practice*. www.gmc-uk.org/guidance/good_medical_practice.asp
Goldacre, B. (2012). *Bad Pharma: How Drug Companies Mislead Doctors and Harm Patients*. London: Fourth Estate.
Gøtzsche, P. (2013). *Deadly Medicines and Organised Crime: How Big Pharma Has Corrupted Healthcare*. London: Radcliffe Publishing LTD.
Gramsci, A. (1971 [1929–1935]). *Selection from the Prison Notebooks*. Q. Hoare and G. Nowell Smith, eds. London: Lawrence & Wishart.
Guillemin, J. (1998). Bioethics and the coming of the corporation to medicine. In R. DeVries and J. Subedi, eds. *Bioethics and Society*. Upper Saddle River, NJ: Prentice Hall, pp. 60–77.
Hawkes, N. (2011). Cameron promotes new partnership between research, industry, and the NHS. *BMJ*, 343, p. d7956.

Hiam, L., Dorling, D., Harrison, D. and McKee, M. (2017). What caused the spike in mortality in England and Wales in January 2015? *Journal of the Royal Society of Medicine*, 110(4), pp. 131–137.

Iglesia, R., ed. (1943). *Historia Verdadera de la Conquista de la Nueva España Vol. II.* Mexico: Secretaría de Educación Popular, p. 394.

Imber, J. (1998). Medical publicity before bioethics: Nineteenth-century illustrations of twentieth-century dilemmas. In R. DeVries and J. Subedi, eds. *Bioethics and Society.* Upper Saddle River, NJ: Prentice Hall, pp. 16–37.

Imber, J. (2008). *Trusting Doctors: The Decline of Moral Authority in American Medicine.* Princeton, NJ: Princeton University Press.

Kassirer, J. (2005). *On the Take: How Medicine's Complicity with Big Business Can Endanger Your Health.* Oxford: Oxford University Press.

Kleinman, A. (1995). Anthropology of bioethics. In A. Kleinman, ed. *Writing at the Margin: Discourse between Anthropology and Medicine.* Berkeley: University of California Press, pp. 41–67.

Koch, T. (2012). *Thieves of Virtue: When Bioethics Stole Medicine.* Cambridge, MA: MIT Press, p. 255.

Koch, T. (2014). The hippocratic thorn in bioethics' hide: Cults, sects, and strangeness. *Journal of Medicine and Philosophy*, 39(1), pp. 75–88.

Kutcher, G. (2009). *Contested Medicine: Cancer Research and the Military.* Chicago: The University of Chicago Press.

Marx, K. (1932 [1846]). *The German Ideology.* www.marxists.org/archive/marx/works/1845/german-ideology/ch01a.htm

Marx, K. (1967). *Capital: A Critique of Political Economy Vol. III: The Process of Capitalist Production as a Whole.* New York: International Publishers, p. 817.

Marx, K. (1969 [1845]). Theses on Feuerbach. In *Marx/Engels Selected Works Vol. I.* Moscow: Progress Publishers, pp. 13–15.

Marx, K. (1990 [1867]). *Capital Volume I.* London: Penguin.

National Institute for Health and care Excellence (2013). *Judging Whether Public Health Interventions Offer Value for Money.* www.nice.org.uk/advice/lgb10/chapter/judging-the-cost-effectiveness-of-public-health-activities

NHS Core Principles (2011). *Principle 4.* www.nhs.uk/nhsengland/thenhs/about/pages/nhscoreprinciples.aspx

Pellegrino, E. (1999). One hundred fifty years later: The moral status and relevance of the AMA Code of Ethics. In Baker et al., 1999, p. 120.

Reiner, R. (2006). Neo-liberalism, crime and criminal justice. *Renewal: A Journal of Labour Politics*, 14(3), pp. 10–22.

Rosenberg, C. (1999). Meanings, policies, and medicine: On the bioethical enterprise and history. *Daedalus*, 128(4), pp. 27–46.

Rothman, D. (2003 [1991]). *Strangers at the Bedside: A History of How Law and Bioethics Transformed Medical Decision Making.* New York: Aldine de Gruyter.

Rubin, E. (1915). *Synsoplevede Figurer.* Copenhagen: Gyldendals.

Shem, S. (1978). *The House of God.* London: Black Swan, p. 19.

Stevens, T. (2000). *Bioethics in America: Origins and Cultural Politics.* Baltimore: Johns Hopkins University Press.

Stewart, A. (2001). *Theories of Power and Domination.* London: Sage, p. 30.

Swedberg, R. (2005). Elective affinities (Wahlverwandtschaften). In *The Max Weber Dictionary: Key Words and Central Concepts.* Stanford, CA: Stanford University Press, pp. 83–84.

Thomas, K. (2017). Trump's F.D.A. pick could undo decades of drug safeguards. *The New York Times*. www.nytimes.com/2017/02/05/health/with-fda-vacancy-trump-sees-chance-to-speed-drugs-to-the-market.html, February 5.

Weber, M. (2011). *The Protestant Ethic and the Spirit of Capitalism*. Oxford: Oxford University Press.

Weiss, J. (2006, November 12). 'Kumbaya': How did a sweet simple song become a mocking metaphor?. *The Dallas Morning News*. www.dallasnews.com/sharedcontent/dws/dn/religion/stories/DN-kumbaya_11rel.ART0.State.Edition1.3e6da2d.html

The World Bank (1993). *World Development Report 1993: Investing in Health*. Oxford: Oxford University Press.

World Medical Association (2006). *WMA Declaration of Geneva*. Divonne-les-Bains, France. www.wma.net/en/30publications/10policies/g1/

World Medical Association (2013). *WMA Declaration of Helsinki – Ethical Principles for Medical Research Involving Human Subjects*. Fortaleza, Brazil. www.wma.net/en/30publications/10policies/b3/

3 Organisational ethics

A solution to the challenges of markets in healthcare?

Lucy Frith

Introduction

The NHS in England is an organisation undergoing substantial change. The passage of the Health and Social Care Act 2012 introduced extensive 'market-style' reforms of the NHS that aimed to encourage new configurations of organisational types providing healthcare (such as commercial companies, social enterprises and charities). These developments could create distinctive ethical issues and sharpens the need for attention to be paid to the ethical operation of healthcare organisations themselves. One solution is to address ethics at an organisational level. This chapter will consider whether organisational ethics programmes could be developed in the UK to address some of the possible ethical issues raised by this new healthcare environment. I will advance a critical analysis of the use of organisational ethics, considering whether it is a conciliatory or emancipatory development and if it can be used to challenge changing conceptions of the role of the NHS.

Health policy in England

Arguably, the biggest, most fundamental changes in the NHS have occurred in the last 30 years, a period when state provision of welfare and goods was questioned and a neo-liberal philosophy of rolling back the state gained greater ascendance (Hunter, 2013). Many diverse policy and social trends have led to the reforms that cannot be fully considered in this chapter (see Dopson, 2009). However, some central claims underpinning the justifications for this move away from the post-war consensus on the welfare state have been articulated by both Labour and Conservative governments. First, the NHS was seen as an inefficient hierarchical monopoly with little accountability that could not contain costs or provide good quality care to patients (Letwin & Redmond, 1988; Le Grand, 2007). Second, the private sector was thought to be better managed and the NHS should learn from this (Mohan, 2009). Third, market forces would encourage leaner more efficient service provision thought competition, which would improve the quality of healthcare and stimulate innovation by ensuring that the best providers were chosen by commissioners and patients (Health Foundation, 2011, Petratos 2018).

The idea of the market as the ideal regulator culminated in the passage of the Health and Social Care Act in 2012. The Act changed how healthcare is commissioned (bought). It established clinical commissioning groups (CCGs) (overseen by NHS England) – who have responsibility for commissioning services for their local populations replacing Primary Care Trusts and Strategic Health Authorities. The 'any qualified provider' initiative, (NHS Confederation, 2011) enabled patients to choose from a range of providers from different sectors: commercial, third sector and the NHS. This built on previous initiatives to encourage non-NHS organisations to bid for services previously offered by the NHS. Section 75 of the 2012 Act, described as the 'engine of privatisation' (Chand, 2013), ensures that NHS contracts are opened up to the market. The regulations state that CCGs must put all services out to tender unless they can prove the service could only be provided by one particular provider. As one commentator notes: 'This reform represents the completion of the roll-out of competition throughout NHS-funded provision' (Reynolds, 2011).

The term commercialisation and 'market' in healthcare are notoriously difficult to define and are often used in multiple, normatively laden ways. Callahan makes a distinction between two kinds of market intervention: those that aim for fundamental change, that include privatisation, moving parts of the system out of government hands; and interventions that aim for market mechanisms to improve efficiency without changing the underlying system (Callahan & Wasunna, 2006). I would argue that the healthcare reforms in the 2012 Act aimed to bring about the first conception of a market in healthcare, building on the previous health reforms that had achieved the latter. This is not a lone view. Many authors have pointed out that these current healthcare reforms will lead to the expansion of commercial providers (Hunter, 2013; McKee et al., 2011). Nonetheless, others such as Rudolf Klein see these changes as part of the continued evolution of the NHS, arguing, 'The NHS in England is being neither privatized nor destroyed' (Klein, 2013).

Markets can vary depending on the mechanisms used to foster competition and choice, who pays for healthcare, how doctors are reimbursed for their services, and how the sector is regulated (Petratos 2018). Powell (2015) advances a 'mixed economy of welfare' perspective that takes a three-dimensional approach to consider different aspects of health systems. This classification can be used to assess how far market mechanisms have penetrated into the NHS: who owns the resource; who finances it; and how it is regulated (Petratos 2018)? First, ownership of the NHS. This still lies largely with the state, but there is increasing provision by non-NHS providers and areas of activity are being transferred to the private sector. The Department of Health has divested in certain areas; for example, in 2013 it sold an 80% share in Plasma Resources UK to Bain Capital, a private equity firm, for £200m (Rankin, 2013). In 2013 NHS Property Services, a limited company owned by the Secretary of State for Health, was set up to manage NHS property and facilities. This company oversees the selling off of NHS property that is deemed surplus to requirements, and acts as a landlord, renting properties back to the NHS organisation – creating another internal market. It has been announced that from the 2016–17 financial year these rents will be charged at market rates. Therefore, assets are being transferred out of the system, and a new form of commercial pressure introduced with some NHS organisations facing rent increases.[1]

Second, who finances healthcare? Although the state still pays for the bulk of health-related expenditure, the use of private sector finance has grown. For example, Public Finance Initiatives (PFI) such as the Local Improvement Finance Trust were introduced in 2000 to improve primary care facilities. These co-financing arrangements are the most profound change in the NHS, as it represents a move towards more private financing of healthcare (Powell & Miller, 2016). Finally, in terms of regulation – arguably this has increased – with the Act extending the role of Monitor, from overseeing foundation trusts, to acting as the oversight body to manage this new competitive environment (merging with the NHS Trust Development Authority in 2015 to become NHS Improvement). NHS England and NHS Improvement now have greater control over providers and commissioners (Ham, 2016), which could be used to keep in check the negative effects of market mechanisms in the NHS. However, as Hunter notes (2013), regulation is often ineffective and cannot be relied upon to keep the system in check. There have been recent policy developments such as the Five Year Forward View (2014) that puts the emphasis on co-operation rather than competition. Hence, how the balance of power between regulators, different types of provider, commissioners and ultimately patients will play out in this changing environment is an area for future study (see Allen et al., 2017).

In sum, 'market' thinking has undoubtedly increased in healthcare policy in England over the last 30 years or so. While keeping the central idea of healthcare free at the point of delivery and, largely, paid for by the state, the main market mechanism that has been introduced in the English NHS is a degree of competition into the supply side of the chain between providers. This form of competition has resulted in new relationships being created between providers and commissioners and new regulatory mechanisms (NHS Improvement and NHS England) to oversee these ways of operating. Part of this is the drive to give patients more choice over providers to increase efficiency, equity and the quality of healthcare (Dixon et al., 2010). The coalition government's white paper, *Liberating the NHS*, which formed the basis of the 2012 Act, set out to give patients more control over their healthcare. This ideological drive to roll back the state, put greater emphasis on consumer choice and prioritise efficiency drives, could ultimately make the state, 'an overseer and purchaser of services rather than their provider' (Greener, 2008). The increasing commercialisation and corporatisation of healthcare is something that has been debated in other disciplines, notably sociology and political philosophy, but relatively little attention has been paid to the ethical aspects of this issue in the UK (Frith, 2013).

1. Ethical aspects of this new environment

The purpose of this chapter is not to debate whether these moves to a more market-orientated healthcare system are, in themselves, a positive or negative development (see Frith, 2016 for an analysis of this debate and Petratos 2018). Whereas Petratos makes the case for further decentralisation, and Epstein (2018) suggests a shift to a humanist medicine, this chapter focusses on what kind of ethical issues might arise in the new healthcare environment and how these might be managed. There are a number of possible ethical concerns that could result from the increasing use of providers outside the NHS. With the increase in private providers, conflicts of interest might be created – such as a conflict between patient welfare and the profitmaking aims of an organisation. A recent debate over the use of 'additional interventions' in IVF fertility treatment illustrates the tensions and perceptions of conflicts of interest when fees are charged for services and provided by commercial organisations in a UK context. Heneghan et al. (2016) published a review of interventions offered in addition to standard IVF and argued that many of these were not evidenced-based. They framed the debate by pointing to the high cost of IVF itself (an area of medicine where 59% is provided privately in the UK) and how these 'add-ons' push the cost up even higher, the implication being they were offered purely for commercial rather than clinical reasons. For my purposes, whether the review makes valid claims about the lack of an evidence-base for some interventions is a side-issue. The key point, as Balen notes, is that,

> Unlike patients with cancer . . . many people are required to self-fund their treatment . . . . The funding landscape was the much needed context missing from the media coverage this week, which conflated evidence-based medicine with treatment costs . . . . It may be true that some clinics are charging for treatments that aren't yet fully proven and this needs to be explained fully to patients.

> (Balen, 2016)

He goes on to say that the central issue is lack of NHS funding for fertility treatment, which means people have to seek treatment in the private sector. While the lack of NHS funding for fertility treatment is not a result of recent health reforms, this example illustrates the kinds of tensions that can arise in a dual system of NHS treatment that sits alongside private provisions.

There is some evidence from the UK to suggest that the more market driven environment is already influencing healthcare delivery. A recent study on the views of nursing staff that had relocated to Independent Sector Treatment Centres (which are private providers of routine and low risk care) from the NHS found that, 'clinicians described new ways of working as extending managerial or corporate control over clinical practice' (Waring & Bishop, 2012). This illustrated 'a production or factory-like model of healthcare . . . . The priority given to productivity was seen by many staff and managers as driven by the need to make the ISTC commercially viable' (Waring, 2015). Some respondents expressed concerns that productivity took precedence over quality of care. One manager said, 'This is a business at the end of the day, we have got to make it work financially' (Waring, 2015). Concepts of professionalism that operate within these private providers are changing (Frith, 2013), with efficiency and performance indicators taking centre stage and the long-term effects on patient care uncertain. This shows some support for the contention that something is lost if medicine becomes subject to the same kinds of commercial ethos and pressures as more market-orientated services.

The system that is evolving will still maintain a large amount of provision by NHS organisations with independent providers bidding for particular services, sometimes in conjunction with NHS organisations. Monitor, now NHS Improvement, the body set up to oversee this new market in healthcare, has three functions: to oversee competition, regulate prices and ensure continuity of care. One possible concern could be the problem of market failure. The 'new' system, in order to stimulate competition, will allow more market failure than in the past. This is a concern, as it is not seen as acceptable if hospitals fail and go out of business. An example of this is Hinchingbrooke Hospital in Cambridgeshire. It was taken over by Circle Healthcare (a private company) in 2011, and they pulled out of the contract in 2015, after it became clear that they had initially submitted an unrealistic bid to win the contract (Scourfield, 2016). Petratos, in his discussion of the 'economic calculation' arguments, points to the benefits of decentralisation[2] and argues that a greater mixed of providers from different sectors can improve the efficiency of healthcare provision. However, the example of Hinchingbrooke Hospital illustrates how market mechanisms are constrained in healthcare (see Frith, 2016, for a discussion of this point). This hospital was taken over by Circle, a private company, and had to be taken back by the NHS when the company pulled out of the contract. Unlike economic operations in other areas, the hospital simply cannot not 'go out of business'. Heath, for example, argues that the most persuasive reason for public provision of healthcare is efficiency. The role of the state is to resolve collective action problems and the welfare state, 'emerges in those areas where liberal markets fail to produce optimal outcomes' (Heath, 2011). Heath argues that the "normative logic" of these [welfare] systems is one of efficiency. This is the 'public-economics' model – the state can provide and finance healthcare more efficiently than if this was left to the market.

Although Monitor has powers to additionally regulate specific services if they are failing, this aspect of competition needs to be balanced against protecting patients (Chand, 2013). With the dual system of provision, how the burden of market failure will effect NHS organisations is a complex issue. As the King's Fund has noted when they considered the effects of these new providers on the local health economy:

> In the current context of substantial cuts in public spending and little or no increase in NHS budgets, any growth in the market share of one organisation is more likely to be at the expense of another organisation. This may result in some existing NHS organisations becoming financially unstable, and difficulties in ensuring seamless care for patients across organisational boundaries.
>
> (King's Fund, 2011)

2. Ways forward – the growth of organisational ethics

There is a growing body of work in 'organisational ethics'. It addresses the ethical attributes and functions of organisations themselves, rather than focussing, as much of bioethics has done to date, on individual relationships (Spencer et al., 2000; Hall,

2000; Gibson et al., 2008). 'Organizational ethics is the study of the ethical behaviour of organizations. It involves clarifying and evaluating the values embedded in organizational policies and practices' (Ellis & Macdonald, 2002). It considers the ethical implications of organisational decisions on key stakeholders, the ethical issues raised by the governance and management and, 'the ethical complexities of balancing the goal of quality patient care with other important goals such as financial sustainability, staff well-being, learning and innovation' (Gibson, 2012). Important questions for study from an organisational ethics perspective are: What are the organisations' alleged aims and values (sometimes contained in a mission statement)? How does the organisation behave ethically in its financial and business arrangements? What are the organisation's work practices, policies, promotion criteria, organisational structures? How does the organisation manage conflicts of interest? What are organisations' duties to their stakeholders? How do the organisation's activities affect the wider community?

The growth in interest in organisational ethics has philosophical roots (Hall, 2000). A focus on the organisation has been claimed to be a natural progression for bioethics, a turn towards an ecological version of bioethics that considers 'the moral sociology of organizations' (Potter, 1996) and the broader context of individuals as biosocial organisms. The interest in organisational ethics was also stimulated by the social and political context of healthcare provision in the U.S. in the late 1980s early 1990s, a period of transition in the organisation of healthcare in the U.S. The development of managed care and the dual responsibilities of healthcare organisations to run as businesses produced fears that healthcare was becoming increasingly commercialised with detrimental effects on patient care (Pearson, Sabin & Emanuel, 2003). There was a perception that money was becoming the dominant focus and traditional moral motives and professionalism were under threat. Mechanic (1996) argued that one of the reasons for the declining trust in the medical profession is the increase in the involvement of for-profit companies in U.S. healthcare. Donald Light argued that marketisation of medicine is the biggest threat to professional knowledge and practice, and that healthcare professionals 'need to be rescued from market forces and from pursuing their own interests' (Light, 2010).

Such concerns over the ethical operation of HCOs were exemplified by the Joint Commission on Accreditation of Healthcare Organizations (JCAHO) (Schyve, 1996) developing standards in 1995 to ensure that hospitals' business practices were conducted ethically. This was a recognition that the boundary between clinical ethics and business ethics can break down in healthcare and business practices need to be subjected to ethical scrutiny in the same way as the doctor-patient relationship in clinical ethics (Schyve, 1996).

3. The relationship between organisational ethics and other 'ethics'

Clinical and professional ethics have a key place in ensuring that practice is conducted ethically. So how do organisational ethics fit into this broader schema? Bean (2011) points to a demarcation between clinical and organisational ethics employed in some of the literature. She argues that a clear line cannot be drawn between organisational and clinical ethics – clinical ethics issues have an organisational dimension and organisational issues will affect patient care and clinical issues. Spencer et al. (2000) also argue that often clinical ethics problems have organisational implications, and they also have an organisational *analogue* – i.e. confidentiality is important at an organisational level, as well as at an individual clinical level. 'Organizational responsibility [for] . . . values cannot be limited to or reduced to their clinical responsibility' (Spencer, 2000:46). They also point to the organisational *causes* of many clinical-ethics problems.

Hence, these two forms of ethics are inextricably related, and it is a matter of hierarchy and focus that differentiates them. Organisational ethics has broad concerns (of which clinical ethics is, probably, the most important element). Hence, it sits at a meso-level to the micro-level of clinical ethics. Organisational ethics focusses on organisational policies, operations, structures and leadership. A key element in thinking about organisational ethics is the recognition that individual healthcare professionals' actions and decision-making take place within a prescribed organisational context – while they can react to this context – the context shapes the options available and how 'appropriate' responses are constructed and delineated. Spencer et al. point out that the construction of this context, the hierarchical structures of the HCO, power relations, finance, personnel issues and the ethical implication of these are often not addressed explicitly by organisations *at all* under any form of ethics or governance and therefore, 'There is a dramatic need for a broader conception of ethics in HCOs' (2000:48).

4. Organisational ethics programmes

So what is an organisational ethics programme? What distinguishes them from other initiatives that are generally seen as part of a clinical ethics programme? There are many practical approaches to instituting clinical ethics into HCOs: the Ethics Liaison Program (Bates et al., 2016) that aims to make ethics part of the moral culture of an institution, The Nijmegen Method, clinical pragmatism (Steinkamp & Gordijn, 2003),[3] and moral case deliberation (Molewijk et al., 2008). These models and methods give guidance and procedures for approaching ethical issues in clinical practice. These initiatives are all valuable and have similar aims to an organisational ethics programme – to improve patient care and experience by supporting staff in their ethical decision-making. However, they do not address the meso-level of ethics: how the organisation functions ethically; the structural elements that set the context in which these clinical ethics issues arise; and how the parameters of action and solutions are constructed.

The IntegratedEthics™ Programme instituted at the Veterans Health Administration in the U.S. (Fox et al., 2010), is an example of a programme that specifically aims to address these organisational issues and integrates ethics at all levels in an organisation. This Programme considers ethics at the level of decisions and actions; systems and processes; and environment and culture. The first level is broadly clinical ethics as usually conceived, such as ethics consultation. The second level is a consideration of the systems and processes that 'create' ethical issues – systemic ethical issues – and seek to prevent such issues arising. The third level is addressing the organisational culture of the organisation by considering how the leadership of an organisation can promote an ethically aware organisation. For instance, performance targets could include ethical dimensions and a culture fostered that promotes and values ethical behaviour and prioritises it as much as organisational efficiency. Thus, this programme is a kind of 'total' ethics approach where *all* ethical aspects of an organisation are covered.

In the UK, we have had less of a tradition of ethics consultants and individual on-site ethics support. The way it has largely developed in the UK is for HCOs to have a clinical ethics committee (CEC). The number of clinical ethics committees is growing, (Slowther et al., 2012) reported an increase from 20 committees in 2001 to 82 in 2010.[4] However, the coverage of these committees is patchy; not all hospitals have them and those that do sometimes report that they are under-utilised. Unlike the U.S. and Canada, there is no regulatory requirement for HCOs in the UK to have an ethics clinical committee. Hence, CECs have developed in an *ad hoc* way, with committees operating with different remits and having different roles within the organisation. Schwartz Rounds, originally developed in the U.S., are a way of supporting staff to provide compassionate care by giving space for reflecting on the emotional and social aspects of their work. These have gained in popularity after the Francis Report in 2013, with 116 organisations instituting these rounds (Robert et al., 2017). However, neither CECs nor Swartz rounds generally address organisational issues, and Swartz Rounds do not focus specifically on the ethical aspects of practice. There is no reason why CECs could not take on a more organisational-ethical role (McClimans et al., 2012). As Slowther et al. (2012) note, CECs largely arose out of clinicians' need for support in making difficult decisions about patient care: 'It is perhaps not surprising that the primary focus of the service was to respond to clinicians rather than the wider hospital community or to patients and families' (p213).

The NHS Institute for Innovation and Improvement's[5] 'Living our Local Values' (LLVs) initiative (2008) is probably the closest thing the NHS has had to an organisational ethics programme. LLVs built on the values set out in the NHS constitution and developed resources to help NHS organisations put these values into practice. The rationale for this was put in the following terms:

> As our healthcare system becomes increasingly devolved, autonomous and entrepreneurial, there is a need for system-wide values, which reaffirm the social purpose of the NHS, to staff, patients and the public and inspire behaviours that put the needs of patients, staff and the public foremost in people's minds.
>
> (II&I, 2008:1)

LLVs put an emphasis on organisational values, processes and leadership, and developed a resource to support HCOs to embed these values throughout the organisation. This was designed to improve the quality of care patients receive, staff experience and public confidence by helping NHS organisations become 'value living' organisations to, 'enable them to sustain change, mobilises collective good will and increase quality and productivity' (II&I, 2008). This was a valuable initiative, but there was no mechanism once the project had finished to ensure its continuation or to evaluate any longer-term outcomes or effects of instituting this work. Today, there a number of trusts who have 'Living our values' initiatives and publish statements of values on their websites. However, just how far these values are embedded and what concrete difference they make to the organisational functioning is a subject for future investigation.

5. Developing organisational ethics in a UK context

Given the changing face of healthcare provisions in England, and its greater focus on competition and patient choice, a closer attention to ethical aspects of organisational functioning is timely. In this section, I want to consider critically if developing organisational ethics programmes in the NHS would be a useful mechanism for addressing the potential ethical issues that might arise in this new environment.

A fundamental question is whether 'ethics' at any level is the best mechanism for addressing the perceived problems and emerging ethical issues created by increased marketisation in the NHS. Many well-known critiques of the bioethics project, often originating from social scientists, see bioethics as empirically uninformed and too led by abstract theory that encourages 'ivory tower' thinking, disconnected from the 'real-world'.[6] A common theme in these critiques is that bioethics is not as critical or as challenging to 'medicine' as either bioethicists think it is or it *should* be. Ivan Illich saw medical ethics as a handmaiden to medicine: 'Medical ethics have been secreted into a specialized department that brings theory into line with actual practice' (Illich, 1976). In his history of bioethics in Britain, Duncan Wilson points out that while bioethics has been portrayed as a radicalising force challenging the medical profession and bringing patients to the fore, others have argued that 'bioethical impulses found their way into enduring social institutions not because they represented the social challenges of the 1960s but because they successfully diffused those challenges' (Stevens, quoted in Wilson, 2012:2). Wilson's account locates the rise of bioethics in the UK as part of 'the neo-liberal demand for oversight whilst also safeguarding medicine' (Wilson, 2011:5). Similarly, Adam Hedgecoe has been critical of bioethics' ability to offer any meaningful criticism of scientific developments in the medical arena. He argues that 'bioethicists accept unquestioningly scientists' expectations about the development of ethical issues . . . and engage in an ethical debate, the boundaries of which have been laid down and defined by academic and industry scientists' (Hedgecoe, 2009:163). Thus, bioethics, from the point of view of this critique, is a socially produced mechanism that is mobilised to fulfil different functions, depending on the context, i.e. control, regulation, legitimation and governance, but rarely offers any radical critique of its objects of study.

It could be claimed that an organisational ethics programme attempts to put certain values at the heart of healthcare at a time when the system has actually moved away from these values. Healthcare provision is no longer seen as a social good, motivated by concerns for the welfare of society, but a commercial enterprise, and the adoption of a more market-orientated model threatens these core values of public service. Illich argued that medicine sought to 'engineer the dreams of reason' and medical ethics legitimised the increasing use of medical technology by focussing the debate on *how* technologies should be employed rather than *if* they should. Correspondingly, it could be argued that organisational ethics provides a legitimate face for a marketised NHS, where *how* the market is rolled out and *how* patients are protected is debated rather than *if* we should move toward this model. Epstein (2018) makes a related critique of medical ethics, arguing that there is, 'a gap between the role the ethic seems to play and the role it actually plays'. Medical ethics is needed by a capitalist medical system to give it the appearance of a humanistic medicine: medical ethics is a part of the very problem it is – ostensibly – trying to solve. Therefore, the role 'ethics' plays in these changes is to reassure and provide a legitimisation of the new trends, rather than critique and challenge.

In this vein, it could be argued that up until now we have had no need to pay attention to organisational ethics, since important core values – such as access and equality – were enshrined in our publicly funded and provided NHS. The NHS Constitution states, 'the NHS should make explicit its values and commitments to patients' (DH, 2013). One of the key principles reads: 'Access to NHS services is based on clinical need, not an individual's ability to pay.' However, David Hunter has argued that core NHS values are under threat:

> Free at the point of delivery is not the only principle invoked . . . . Bevan's principles were also about the way things are delivered . . . . This is a critical point because many of those who ostensibly support the NHS view it principally as a funding mechanism rather than as the deliverer of care services which, they believe, could just as well (or better) be undertaken by a range of for-profit and not-for-profit bodies as well as public ones.
>
> (Hunter, in the Bevan Commission, 2011)

Therefore, the increase in non-NHS providers is a challenge to the original conception of the NHS – that healthcare was state funded *and* state provided. The NHS Constitution also states that 'The NHS belongs to the people.' In this way, a system increasingly characterised by delivery from outside providers, PFI initiatives and disinvestment by the Department of Health shifts the ownership of the NHS away from the state. Hence, this is arguably, from Bevan's core principles. Consequently, I would argue that the increasing marketisation of the NHS does pose new and different ethical challenges for the NHS that need to be addressed at an organisational level.

The development of organisational ethics both in the literature and in practice has, to date, been largely a North American phenomenon. But there are differences between HCOs in the U.S. and the UK. As Ashcroft & Dixon-Woods (2011) note, it is impossible to underestimate the importance of the NHS as a public service, administered by central government and accountable to parliament and the electorate, as well as the courts, professional bodies, and patients. Thus, problems that in the U.S. system and elsewhere may be handled as local issues of quality or performance arising in a network of private actors (HMOs, hospitals, state medical boards individual doctors), can, in the U.K., become political problems very quickly, and very potently.

(pp. 81–2)

This points to key differences in the context of HCOs in the UK and the U.S. The NHS is arguably in one respect a discrete organisation in its own right, with its own policies, regulations and guidelines that pertain across individual HCOs. Thus, organisational ethics programmes instituted in individual organisations might be limited in the scope of what they can achieve. A pan-NHS organisational ethics programme, run from NHS England for example, might better serve organisational ethics in a NHS context. This could be based on professional values, legal principles of equality, equity and access and principles underpinning the NHS set out in the NHS constitution for example. While this may be a goal to aim for, organisational ethics programmes at individual HCO level can still play a useful role. In the current climate we are moving towards more autonomous Trusts, more non-NHS providers, health devolution (in Manchester) and greater fragmentation, with the role of central NHS oversight decreasing. Therefore, ethics at a local level could become more important.

6. Critical organisational ethics

In order to address some of the above critiques and to advance an organisational ethics that does not become a 'handmaiden' to existing power structures, we need to develop a 'critical organisational ethics'. The term 'critical' has been used in social science to delineate types of scholarship that are critical of particular social practices, such as racism, homophobia etc. Previously seen as 'radical' research, it takes issue with social practices, rather than simply describing or trying to understand them. However, as Andrew Sayer has argued on a number of occasions,

> critical social science, . . . has either become increasingly reticent about making its critiques and their standpoints or rationales explicit, or has softened its critiques, so that in some quarters being critical has reduced to trying merely to "unsettle" some ideas or to being reflexive.
>
> (Olson & Sayer, 2009:181)

The solution to this, for Sayer, is to move towards more normative analysis in social science, recognising that ethics can be discussed 'rationally' and progress made (Sayer, 2011). Bioethics, on the other hand, as noted above, has been accused of the opposite problem, neglecting the social context of its theories and problems. Critical bioethics (for example Hedgecoe, 2004; Murray & Holmes, 2009) often begin by stressing that bioethics needs to embrace a more sociological under-standing of its endeavours and the 'locatedness' of its arguments. Organisational ethics, coming from the discipline of bioethics, has a clear normative focus and the disciplinary tools to address explicitly the 'critical' that Sayer sees as lacking critical social science. This needs to be supplemented by embracing some of the concerns central to the social sciences (locating issues within their socio-cultural context), while recognising bioethics' inherent strength in addressing the norma-tive. Extending the traditional focus of medical ethics, to considering power rela-tions, the socially situated nature of organisations and their decisions and paying particular attention to how actors are embedded in these social contexts – could address the criticisms levied at medical ethics by authors such as Illich and Epstein.

For a critical organisational ethics, these socio-cultural elements could include: empirically informed ethical analysis; a recognition of the social context of HCOs and the power structures that operate both within and outside HCOs; and a broader conception of stakeholder involvement – involving all staff, patients and the wider community and public – to ensure that HCOs operate in the best interests of the whole community and to determine what these best interests might look like. Adding these elements could give a more critical and reflective perspective to organisational ethics programmes and the theoretical discussions over ethics at this level. While these are standard elements in any 'critical bioethics', I argue that organisational ethics needs to be further supplemented by drawing on the theoretical developments in organisational studies to understand change, agency and power at an organisational and systems level. As Currie et al. (2012) have argued, there is a need for a 'positive inter-disciplinary interaction, a "generative dance", between organization studies (OS), and . . . health policy and medical sociology' to better understand contemporary healthcare both theoretically and empirically. This should also be supplemented by organisational ethics, so that the normative implications can be fully theorised. Organisational ethics can join this 'inter-disciplinary genera-tive dance'. It can contribute to a different understanding of HCOs and give guid-ance and insight into the appropriate goals of HCOs and their policies and practices. Most importantly, a critical organisational ethics informed by medical sociology, health policy and organisational studies has the tools to advance a critical perspec-tive on modern HCOs that is sorely often lacking in recent debates.

This critical organisational ethics would differ from existing ethics support mechanisms, as outlined earlier, and it would differ from other forms of 'ethics'. It would attend to the broader social and political context of healthcare, foreground-ing a more sociological understanding that pays attention to power relations, to those who are served well by the system and in whose interests it operates. A pos-sible limitation of the practical application of organisational ethics, in the form of a programme, is that as it has to, by necessity, operate within the organisation and with the organisation's blessing. Therefore, if it invariably becomes an insider, how will it be able to advance a critical perspective? The following elements could address this issue, and it is one that all organisational ethics programmes have to address. First, a robust area of research on critical organisational ethics could provide a basis for showing how practice has changed in other areas and providing some 'outsider' perspectives to aid internal change. Second, the involvement of a wider range of stakeholders, particularly the public, users and patients, would mean that a wider range of views are heard. Finally, in an NHS context, it is possible that organisational ethics programmes need to be constituted at a trans-organisational level, so that there can be a genuine critique of organisations.

7. Conclusions

I argue that organisational ethics programmes could play a role in this new healthcare environment in the NHS in England. Such programmes alone cannot ensure ethical practice, but they can begin to highlight the importance of the ethical aspects of an organisation's operation. The ethical dimensions of these new organisational forms, new provider relationships and a health sector that combines public and private provision should not be ignored.

Notes

1 See NHS Property website www.property.nhs.uk/ and a discussion of their operations by the National Audit Committee (2014).
2 The NHS has long grappled with the tensions of trying to provide a decentralised local service, while also having direction and control from the centre in the form of the Department of Health; see Klein (2013).
3 See this paper for an overview of four methods of ethical case deliberation (clinical pragmatism, The Nijmegen Method, hermeneutic and Socratic dialogue).
4 According to the UK Clinical Ethics Network website, there are now 83 ethics committees registered with the Network.
5 This body was replaced in 2013 by NHS Improving Quality, which has now become The Sustainable Improvement Team.
6 There are counters to these critiques; see Turner (2009) for a good summary of some of the shortcomings of the social science critique.

References

Allen, P. et al. (2017) Commissioning through competition and cooperation in the English NHS under the Health and Social Care Act 2012: Evidence from a qualitative study of four local health economies. *BMJ Open,* 7: e011745. doi:10.1136/bmjopen-2016-011745

Ashcroft, R. & Dixon-Woods, M. (2011) The social forms and functions of bioethics in the United Kingdom. In: Myser, C. (ed.) *Bioethics Round the Globe.* Oxford: Oxford University Press pp. 76–92.

Balen, A. (2016) IVF practices challenged? www.adambalen.com/ivf-practices-challenged-2/

Bates, S. et al. (2016) The ethics liaison program: Building a moral community. *Journal of Medical Ethics,* 43: 595-600. doi: 10.1136/medethics-2016–103549

Bean, S. (2011) Navigating the murky intersection between clinical and organizational ethics: A hybrid case taxonomy. *Bioethics,* 25, 6: 320–325.

The Bevan Commission (2011) Are Bevan's principles still applicable in the NHS? Improving Healthcare White Paper Series – No. 3. www.1000livesplus.wales.nhs.uk/sitesplus/documents/1011/Are%20Bevans%20Principles%20White%20Paper.pdf

Callahan, D. & Wasunna, A. (2006) *Medicine and the Market: Equity v. Choice*. Baltimore: The John Hopkins University Press.

Chand, K. (2013) NHS: Section 75 of the health act is an engine for destruction. *The Guardian*. www.theguardian.com/commentisfree/2013/apr/22/section-75-health-act-destruction-engine

Currie, G. et al. (2012) Let's dance: Organization studies, medical sociology and health policy. *Social Science & Medicine*, 74: 273–280.

Department of Health (2009) *NHS Constitution*. London: DH (revised 2013).

Dixon, A. et al. (2010) Patient choice: How patients choose and how providers respond. *The Kings Fund*. www.kingsfund.org.uk/sites/files/kf/Patient-choice-final-report-Kings-Fund-Anna_Dixon-Ruth-Robertson-John-Appleby-Peter-Purge-Nancy-Devlin-Helen-Magee-June-2010.pdf

Dopson, S. (2009) Changing forms of managerialism in the NHS: Hierarchies, markets and networks. In Gabe, J. & Calnan, M. (eds.), *The New Sociology of the Health Service*. London: Routledge. pp. 37–55.

Ellis, C. & Macdonald, C. (2002, Fall) Implications of organizational ethics to healthcare. *Healthcare Management Forum*, 15, 3: 32–38.

Epstein, M. (2018). The corruption of medical morality under advanced capitalism. In: Feiler, T., Hordern, J. & Papanikitas, A. (eds.), *Marketisation, Ethics and Healthcare: Policy, Practice and Moral Formation*. Abingdon: Routledge. pp. 32–48.

Fox, E., Bottrell, M., Berkowitz, K., et al. (2010) Integrated ethics: An innovative program to improve ethics quality in healthcare. *The Innovation Journal*, 15: 1–36.

Frith, L. (2013) The NHS and Market Forces in healthcare: The need for organisational ethics. *Journal of Medical Ethics*, 39: 17–21.

Frith, L. (2016) The changing face of the English National Health Service: New providers, markets and morality. *British Medical Bulletin*, 119, 1: 5–16.

Gibson, J., Sibbald, R., Connolly, E., et al. (2008) Organizational ethics. In Singer, P. & Viens, A. (eds.), *The Cambridge Textbook of Bioethics*. Cambridge: Cambridge University Press. pp. 243–50.

Gibson, L. (2012, Spring) Organizational ethics: No longer the elephant in the room. *Healthcare Management Forum*, 25, 1: 37–39.

Greener, I. (2008) Markets in the public sector: When do they work, and what do we do when they don't? *Policy and Politics*, 36, 1: 93–108.

Hall, R. (2000) *An Introduction to Healthcare Organizational Ethics*, Oxford: Oxford University Press.

Ham, C. (2016) Government and national bodies take charge of decision making as NHS crisis grows. *BMJ*, 352: i658. doi: 10.1136/bmj.i658

Health Foundation (2011) Competition in Healthcare. www.health.org.uk/sites/health/files/CompetitionInHealthcare.pdf

Heath, J. (2011) Three normative models of the welfare state. *Public Reason*, 3, 2: 13–43.

Hedgecoe, A. (2004) Critical bioethics: Beyond the social science critique of applied ethics. *Bioethics*, 18, 2: 120–143.

Hedgecoe, A. (2010) Bioethics and the reinforcement of socio-technical expectations. *Social Studies in Science*, 40, 2: 163–186.

Heneghan, C. et al. (2016) Lack of evidence for interventions offered in UK fertility Centres. *BMJ*, 355: i6295. doi: 10.1136/bmj.i6295

Hunter, D. (2013) A response to Rudolf Klein. *Journal of Health Politics, Policy and Law*, 38, 4: 871–877.

Illich, I. (1976) *The Limits to Medicine: Medical Nemesis – The Expropriation of Health.* London: Marion Boyers.

Institute for Innovation and Improvement (2008) Living our local values. NHS. http://marymurtaghmedia.co.uk/NHS-The-Value-of-Values.pdf

Kings Fund (2011) Understanding new labour's market reforms of the English NHS. www.kingsfund.org.uk/publications/understanding-new-labours-market-reforms-english-nhs

Klein, R. (2013) The twenty-year war over England's national health service: A report from the battlefield. *Journal of Health Politics, Policy and Law*, 38, 4: 849–869.

Le Grand, J. (2007) *The Other Invisible Hand: Delivering Public Services through Choice and Competition*, Princeton, NJ: Princeton University Press.

Letwin, O. & Redmond, J. (1988) Britain's biggest enterprise: Ideas for reform of the NHS. www.scribd.com/doc/56986348/Britain-s-Biggest-Enterprise

Light, D. (2010) Healthcare professionals, markets and countervailing powers. In Bird, C. (ed.), *Handbook of Medical Sociology*. Vanderbilt University Press. pp. 270–289.

McClimans, L., Slowther, A.-M. & Parker, M. (2012) Can UK clinical ethics committees improve quality of care? *HEC Forum*, 24, 2: 139–47. doi: 10.1007/s10730–012–9175-z

McKee, M. et al. (2011) In defence of the NHS: Why writing to the House of Lords was necessary. *BMJ*, 343: d6535. doi: 10.1136/bmj.d6535

Mechanic, D. (1996) Changing medical organization and the erosion of trust. *Millbank Quarterly*, 74, 2: 171–189.

Mohan, J. (2009) Visions of privatization: New labour and the reconstruction of the NHS. In Gabe, J. & Calnan, M. (eds.), *The New Sociology of the Health Service*. London: Routledge. pp. 79–98.

Molewijk, B. et al. (2008) Teaching ethics in the clinic: The theory and practice of moral case deliberation. *Journal of Medical Ethics*, 34: 120–124.

Murray, S. & Holmes, D. (eds.) (2009) *Critical Interventions in the Ethics of Healthcare.* Abingdon: Routledge.

National Audit Office (2014) Investigation into NHS Property Services Limited. www.nao.org.uk/report/investigation-nhs-property-services-limited/

NHS (2012) *Report on the Effect of the NHS Constitution*. London: DH.

NHS Confederation (2011, July) Any qualified provider. Discussion paper, Issue 10. www.labournet.net/ukunion/1107/Any_qualified_provider.pdf

NHS England. Five Year Forward View. 2014. www.england.nhs.uk/wp-content/uploads/2014/10/5yfv-web.pdf

Olson, E. & Sayer, A. (2009) Radical geography and its critical standpoints: Embracing the normative. *Antipode*, 41, 1: 180–198.

Pearson, S., Sabin, J. & Emanuel, E. (2003) *No Margin, No Mission: Health Organizations and the Quest for Ethical Excellence*. Oxford: Oxford University Press.

Petratos, P. (2018) Why the economic calculation debate matters: the case for decentralisation in healthcare. In Feiler, T., Hordern, J. & Papanikitas, A. (eds.), *Marketisation, Ethics and Healthcare: Policy, Practice and Moral Formation*. Abingdon: Routledge, pp. 13–31.

Potter, R. (1996) From clinical ethics to organisational ethics: The second stage of the evolution of bioethics. *Bioethics Forum*, 12: 3–12.

Powell, M. (2015) Making markets in the English National Health Service. *Social Policy and Administration*, 49, 1: 109–127.

Powell, M. & Miller, R. (2016) Seventy years of privatising the English National Health Service? *Social Policy and Administration*, 50, 1: 99–118.

Rankin, J. (2013) Bain capital buys majority stake in plasma resources UK. *The Guardian.* www.theguardian.com/business/2013/jul/18/bain-capital-plasma-resources-uk

Reynolds, L. (2011) Issues MPs and the media have missed in Lansley's bill. *BMJ*, 342: d3194.

Robert, G. et al. (2017) Exploring the adoption of Schwartz center rounds as an organisational innovation to improve staff well-being in England, 2009–2015. *BMJ Open*, 7: e014326. doi: 10.1136/bmjopen-2016–014326

Sayer, A. (2011) *Why Things Matter to People: Social Science, Values and Ethical Life.* Cambridge: Cambridge University Press.

Schyve, P. (1996) Patient rights and organizational ethics: The joint commission perspective. *Bioethics Forum*, 12: 13–20.

Scourfield, P. (2016) Squaring the circle: What lessons can be learned from the Hinchingbrooke franchise fiasco? *Critical Social Policy*, 36, 1: 142–152.

Slowther, A. et al. (2012) Development of clinical ethics services in the UK: A national survey. *Journal of Medical Ethics*, 38: 210e214. doi:10.1136/medethics-2011–100173

Spencer, E., Mills, A., Rorty, M., et al. (2000) *Organizational Ethics in Healthcare*. Oxford: Oxford University Press.

Steinkamp, N. & Gordijn, B. (2003) Ethical case deliberation on the ward: A comparison of four methods. *Medicine, Healthcare and Philosophy*, 6: 235–246.

Turner, L. (2009) Anthropological and sociological critiques of bioethics. *Bioethical Inquiry*, 6: 83–98.

Waring, J. (2015) Mapping the diaspora. *Public Administration*, 93, 2: 345–362.

Waring, J. & Bishop, S. (2012) Going private: Clinicians experience of working in UK independent sector treatment centres. *Health Policy*, 104: 172–178.

Wilson, D. (2012) Who guards the guardians? Ian Kennedy, bioethics and the 'ideology of accountability' in British medicine. *Social History of Medicine,* 25, 1: 193–211. doi: 10.1093/shm/hkr090

Part II
The influence of the market

4   Encoding truths? Diagnosis-Related Groups and the fragility of the marketisation discourse

Therese Feiler

Introduction[1]

Organisational reforms in healthcare are usually left to economists, public law scholars or social scientists. Intentionally or not, decision-making at the policy-level often converts far-reaching decisions into technocratic jargon. Theologians have been somewhat on the margins of these debates. This is perhaps no surprise, considering the seemingly neutral focus on empirical measures typical of the discourse. Moreover, theological ethics are frequently limited to neuralgic issues such as euthanasia or preimplantation diagnostics. Nonetheless, the marketisation of healthcare has a theological dimension, also at the policy-level.

This chapter will take as an example a particular change in healthcare financing at the meso-level: Diagnosis-Related Groups. DRGs marked a shift in the way hospitals were oriented and were the means to operationalise the market-logic in healthcare. The DRG system is a case classification system: each hospital case is related to a 'pre-standardised product' of treatment. Depending on how a patient's case is encoded, the hospital is reimbursed for the services provided. In this way, hospital care can be matched with pre-calculated resources. Case volumes can be predetermined according to the profit needs of a hospital and an economy's 'healthcare sector' as a whole. Developed in the early 1980s by Robert B. Fetter and John D. Thompson, a management and a public health scholar at Yale, DRGs were first introduced in New Jersey, and have become the key accounting system throughout Western and increasingly LMI countries' healthcare systems. (Mathauer and Wittenbecher 2013) Here I will particularly draw on examples from Germany, Switzerland and Scandinavia, but also to the NHS in England.

What follows is what one might call accompanying research, albeit in a counterpoint movement (Ramsey 2016). The aim is to critically illuminate the theological structures of (sub-)systems such as the DRG. Four constitutive claims will be contested. First, the claim that marketisation is theologically neutral, inherent in the 'clean' language of 'modernisation' reforms. Rather, I argue, it is theologically grounded and implies theological interpretations of how acts of care should relate to political-economic structures; theology itself is a critical heuristic for different systemic challenges. Second, the adjacent assumption that marketisation is a natural, impersonal and global evolution will be contested. In contrast, the meaningful nature of human history makes both individual and systemic responsibility possible in the first place. Third, I will contest the claim that DRGs better represent care. The codification and thus distortion of care raises the question of whether and how to represent it truthfully. It will be suggested that meaningful representation has to *follow* the event, rather than quench it out. Finally, against the claim that DRGs do not touch the substance of medical care, DRGs have in fact challenged the integrity of the medical profession, because they institutionalised contradictory 'logics' of action – medical as opposed to managerial-economic. This invites reflection on the meaning of vocation as an irreducible aspect to the human being and medical practice. These four theological counterpoints to the DRG system – theological significance, historical-systemic responsibility, representation and vocation – destabilise the marketisation discourse exemplified by the DRG system, relocate it and raise the stakes of the debate.

1. *The patient follows the money*: marketisation as theological shift and transvaluation

DRGs classify clinical cases according to several variables: principal and secondary diagnoses, patient age and sex, the presence of co-morbidities and complications, and the procedures performed. Depending on how the clinical case is then coded, reimbursement for each delivered pre-standardised "product" is released to the hospital by payers such as statutory health insurances, Medicare, private insurers, or Clinical Commissioning Groups. In the NHS, for example, operations are coded using the Office of Population, Censuses and Surveys Classification of Surgical Operations and Procedures (OPCS) system. These operation codes, together with diagnostic codes such as the ICD-10, are then converted to generate Healthcare Resource Group (HRG) codes, the English version of DRGs. In the system of "Payment by Results" (PbR) they generate the tariff for reimbursement to the Trust (Department of Health 2013). In the NHS, as in other systems, DRGs have remained one hospital financing mechanism besides others such as block grants, per capita payments and public investment. And whereas block grants are arguably on the state end of the spectrum of financing mechanisms, DRGs or 'activity-based funding' are on the market end, putting a price on each activity (Marshall et al. 2014).

The great selling-point of DRGs was that they were to allow 'money to follow the patient' (OECD 2004; Kimberly et al. 2008; Busse et al. 2011). This almost mythical phrase alludes to the familiar idea that patients are ends in themselves, which translates into 'patient-centredness', 'patient choice' and focus on 'outcomes'. However, because of their *prospective* nature, DRGs pre-determine the categories into which both patients and doctors must fall. As a 'currency' they are used for budget projection and rationalisation to increase 'efficiency' and, or, profits. Targets for activities and volumes are set in advance; bonus payments to clinicians can be related to pre-agreed numbers of cases in a given time-interval, irrespective of patients' actual needs. In this industrial model of contracted 'instances of care', payment is released according to specific numbers of coded cases. Unless the system is gamed to their advantage, the coding thus determines how patients are treated. In other words: *The patient has to follow the money.*

For this reason, DRG reforms were a fundamental, paradigmatic shift, 'the largest and most thoroughgoing reforms of financing, but also of perspectives, of working and acting in the healthcare system' (Braun 2014, p. 91, also Bode 2011). It consists both in the relocation of the patient into a market logic, and the simultaneous redefinition of the patient as consumer-citizen which *conceals* this relocation: we now talk of consumer-clients, healthcare "delivery", instances of care that can be traded, scaled up, etc. The new definition of healthcare, its logic and *telos*, amounts to a 'transvaluation' (*Umwertung*), to use a Nietzschean term.[2] This was operationalised, amongst others, through DRGs.

1.1 Theology and the nature of the healthcare system

There are several starting points for a theological consideration of this development. First, the *historical* project unearths the genealogy of the market as we know it (see also below). Max Weber and Richard H. Tawney recognised the religious presuppositions of industrial capitalism, but more recently also several theologians (Kidwell and Doherty 2015; Skidelsky 2015). Both with and against sociology they have pointed at the Calvinist heritage of 'inner-worldly ascetics', for whom making money was a *religious* vocation. In one contemporary Anglo-Catholic interpretation, the Reformation's emphasis primarily on a person's faith led to a 'dis-connection of reality' from God: bared of all intrinsic justice and good end(s), the world became 'an arbitrary set of disconnected things' (Milbank 2015) and the market an exchange of mere 'stuff'. Whether the Reformation is to blame in this way must be contested. Either way, the market is theologically conditioned.

Conversely, organisational structures of healthcare have been an intrinsic part of the Church's reflection on its service to others (*diakonía*) as a 'fruit of faith' (Turre 1991). In the Middle Ages an aspect of charitable endowments and the monasteries' work, care for the sick was significantly re-ordered in the course of the Reformation. And whilst the Lutheran strand increasingly tasked the state with the provision of public healthcare, the Calvinist tradition embraced a more entrepreneurial model. In the nineteenth and early twentieth centuries, besides the socialist movement, Lutheran as well as Catholic social ethics played an important role in the institution of the modern welfare state. These 'religious schemes of interpretation' continue to 'format what one can call invisible social policy' as well as 'the non-economic foundations of economic action'. They undergird the different models of healthcare provision until today. 'To put it poignantly,' writes Gerhard Wegner, 'neoliberalism then would be the Calvinists' belated revenge on the Wittenbergians' (Wegner 2015, pp. 18–19).

Second, in line with this historical-theological continuum, there is a persistent systematic-theological aspect to the relationship between care for the sick and the market. It touches upon the grounds of the welfare state as that which has traditionally mediated between the two. As Zimmermann-Acklin has pointed out (2010, p. 110), there is now a significant 'contextual gap' between theological reflection and the modern welfare state, despite their shared history. Some theologians mediate this gap by adopting the language of human and constitutional rights or shared concepts of human dignity. Others have traditionally sought to corrode it by reference to natural law (the more Catholic approach) and its principles of solidarity, subsidiarity and personhood. Schnabl, for example, writes: '*Solidarity* transforms the content of neighbour love into the field of the structural and the institutional. With this, a central ethical content of the Jewish-Christian tradition is spelled out into a sphere which in modernity can precisely no longer be developed' (Schnabl cit. in Zimmermann-Acklin 2010, p. 113). This is an admittedly 'reduced theology', in which faith easily shrinks down to a mere individual motivation, but the religious substance remains latent.

Third, this invites a reference to the *sui generis* theological debate around the being and nature of God in relation to the world. This debate sets the premises for the considerations just mentioned. In the light of this meta-narrative, historical and systematic forms can be analysed. In other words, theology functions as a heuristic for the *logic* of healthcare and economics, their modern relationship, and the nature of that debate. Reference may be made to the divine economy of grace, which is presented as profoundly *uneconomical*. Creation, redemption and the new creation are acts of divine generosity (Exod. 3:7–8b). This economy is at work in the liberation both from economic slavery ("the house of bondage", Exod. 20:2; Deut. 5:6, 7–21) and from egotistical desires ("And he died for all, that those who live might live no longer for themselves but for him who for their sake died and was raised" [1 Cor. 5:14–15]).

This uneconomical logic recurs in scriptural passages on material wealth. Proverbs, for example, appreciates wealth, albeit in the context of wisdom (Prov 11:4). Ezekiel meets the market in the context of critical suspicion to the point of hostility. The prophetic thread continues in the New Testament, where the impending divine kingdom engenders an acute, if not disturbing, rejection of material goods and economic considerations (Mark 10:25; Mt 19:24; Lk 18:25). Salvation through the cross would be interpreted as an uneconomically economic event: according to Anselm of Canterbury's theory of atonement, Christ made a restitutive 'payment' to God. The infinite debt owed as a result of human transgression against an infinite God, so the understanding, could only be paid with the sacrificial death of a God-man. Through faith, infinite divine judgment would be avoided. Thus the participation of faith in this divine plenitude was to overcome the economy of transgression, debt and repayment (Bell 2005; Benjamin 1991).

Over against the logic of the market – managing scarcity in the light of conflicting interests – divine plenitude, existence as such, suggests a strong logical, and possibly ontological primacy of nurture and care; reconciliation is understood as *healing*. Not least the parable of the Good Samaritan indicates compassion in principle encompasses everyone rather than a merely contractually founded society (Zimmermann-Acklin 2010, p. 117). Hence the market requires significant boundaries, reorientation and redefinition; it cannot determine its own ends. In every case, the above juxtaposition avoids, and even polemicises against the absolute conflation of the late capitalist market logic and that of healthcare. Even more so since this conflation effectively amounts to the *separation* and *silencing* of genuine healthcare from the managerial health economy. Care for its own sake becomes a subjective motivation, a 'black box' (Powell cit. in Bode and Vogd 2016, p. 9) or an ideologically imposed fiction, threatening with its 'moraline-acidic' paternalism (Patzen 2010; Savulescu and Schuklenk 2017).

Since the early nineteenth century the main churches have continuously wrestled with their relegation to pure internal subjectivity. Recent scholars have set ecclesial practice as a counter-corporation against managerialism and market corporations (Long et al. 2007). This does not necessarily suggest the uneconomic logic of gift may fully replace economic systems. But a horizon of plenitudinous gift that is existence as such is the ground for solidary, diaconic forms of healthcare here. It also inserts significant *doubt* into any healthcare system that is a) based on the maximisation of individual utility, b) is oriented towards – or happens to result in – the mere upwards-moving extraction of profit, and that c) redefines all aspects of healthcare to that effect. Such doubt is particularly strong in healthcare, which addresses the loss and scarcity of physical suffering, often correlated with economic disadvantage and loss.

In the U.S., Scandinavia and Germany, increasingly privatised hospitals certainly have used DRGs to maximise their income, often at the cost of patients. Strategies associated with DRGs include e.g. the 'cream-skimming' of patients with particularly lucrative conditions. This has resulted in unnecessary invasive procedures, but also multiple re-admissions after "bloody" hospital discharges (i.e. before patients had recovered), as well as the relative neglect of patients with chronic diseases. Setting targets through DRGs for particular treatments allowed for an artificial increase or decline in the number of financially rewarding cases. DRGs have also been used to generate hospital income by either making use of the codes' flexibility ('DRG-creep', upcoding or upgrading) or by straightforward fraudulent coding at large scales (Neby et al. 2015; Balleisen 2017, p. 365). The Payment-by-Results system in the NHS 'relies on honesty and transparency between commissioners and providers of clinical services, both working on behalf of patients and in their best interests' (Chambers et al. 2010). But there are no grounds for romanticising the NHS: like others, it is under 'pressures to cook the books' (Cooper 2016, cp. Brennan et al. 2012).

2. Marketisation: 'natural evolution' and systemic (ir)responsibility

A previous point – the possibility that marketisation is just something that happens – is particularly pertinent to the global narrative of New Public Management (NPM) reforms in general and the DRG in particular. This narrative makes frequent reference to impersonal, naturalistic images: the new 'landscape' of healthcare, the organisational 'environment' that is 'emerging'. The OECD consistently presented DRGs as a global development, the natural thrust of progressive modernisation in the face of objective necessities. This language also pervades critical assessments, e.g. when Ingo Bode talks about a 'maelstrom of evolutionary processes' (Bode and Vogd 2016, p. 6). Such imagery chimes with neoliberal thought, which the late Duncan B. Forrester (1997) explored in a useful study of Friedrich A. von Hayek's work. Forrester's analysis illuminates the ahistoricity and the ensuing lack of political responsibility inherent in marketisation, which also explains its resilience in the face of countervailing evidence. This will prompt the second theological counterpoint: history as meaningfully structured.

Hayek distinguishes between two kinds of orders: first, 'contrived orders', devised by humans to serve their purposes. This is what the Greeks called *taxis*, and is illustrated by a line of battle in which the individual is no longer free but under orders. Contrived orders are distinct from 'spontaneous orders', organic growths that are not the result of human planning, decision or calculation. Hayek (1982, cit. in Forrester 1997) calls these the *kosmos*, 'orderly structures which are the product of the action of many men but are not the result of human design' (p. 143). Forrester points out: 'A spontaneous order has no purpose, no *telos*; it has not been brought into being by an outside agency . . . it has "just growed"' (p. 143). Hayek understood the market as such a spontaneous order, the only one in which individuals could freely pursue their interests, goals and purposes. The market, according to Hayek, is '"an impersonal process which brings about a greater satisfaction of human desires than any deliberate human organization could achieve"' (p. 143). Forrester highlights that Hayek adopts the term *catallaxy* for the market order. The word certainly invokes a form of exchange, but Hayek also welcomes connotations of 'to admit into community' and 'to turn from enemy into friend'. He effectively mirrors, and partly parodies, Hobbes' *Leviathan*, the powerful state that stifles the civil war always lurking just under the surface. However nuanced their collusion, then, market and state remain profoundly at odds with theologies of plenitude and teleology.

The ahistorical nature of Hayek's market warrants further attention. It is no coincidence that marketisation gained steam from the 1990s onwards, when Francis Fukuyama famously declared the 'end of history'. From a systematic-theological perspective, the God that acts in history markedly contrasts with the idea that a spontaneously emerging *catallaxy* remains unaffected by conveniently pluralistic human values. The nature of God's interactions with Israel as *historical* is already part of early Israelite faith. Though now virtually impossible to historically reconstruct, early biblical 'original stories' are repeatedly commemorated: biblical narration itself largely consists of repetition, remembering and retelling earlier material. Historical political events are *theologically* interpreted throughout later writings (e.g. the fall of Judah as divine judgement on Israel's sin in the prophets). In the New Testament, the events around Jesus of Nazareth are located in a specific time and space, i.e. first-century Palestine. 'Here history becomes serious, without being sanctified' (Bonhoeffer 2009, p. 104). Up until the Enlightenment, the Bible was a key to world history; the differentiation between profane history and salvation history dates from that era. Their relationship certainly resists homogeneity both in the Bible and contemporary debate. Yet whilst the Bible without history is prone to become simplified and ideologised so any human, culturally meaningful institution requires the horizon of history (Frey et al. 2009, p. xxii). Put differently, for any institution to be legitimate, history itself must be meaningful; this sense is perhaps a residue of history-as-salvation history (Schaper 2009; Milbank 2015). Retelling the history of marketisation, and DRGs in particular, is to understand it as part of our social, political and cultural negotiations, which are hardly bound by the determinism of a brute nature.

As for the DRGs, before they were introduced, hospital financing was largely framed by political structures. Whilst negotiation skills were certainly required of hospital managers, elected politicians were held accountable for budget decisions. Hospitals received their funding for the treatment given to patients, covering *retrospectively* the costs incurred. A frequent complaint about this system was that it led to lengthy stays in hospitals for lack of incentives to discharge patients swiftly, longer waiting lists and, consequently, altogether fewer hospital admissions. The argument was that this keeps "activity" low. But already this argument was part of the cultural drive to (re-)turn healthcare into an economic 'sector' and, in the U.S., to reverse the post-war settlement (Gaffney 2014; Chilingerian 2008). DRGs spread with the varying political champions of healthcare marketisation, such as Reagan in the U.S., Thatcher in the UK, or the Social Democrats in Germany. In Greece and Ireland, they were adopted as late as 2013 and 2014 as part of the European budget discipline (under German oversight) in the wake of the financial crisis (Burke et al. 2016). Yet these events require interpretation, locating the interpreter and his future possibilities. Hence, *history* marks a significant counterpoint to the natural-evolutionary imagery accompanying marketisation. In the remembrance of alternatives, history functions as a depository of freedom.

2.1 Systemic (ir)responsibility

On the back of the market as an ahistorical order, Hayek effectively limits systemic, political responsibility for a just social order, which makes Petratos' (2018) neat allocation of responsibilities in the present volume difficult to sustain. Hayek does assume that justice exists as an objective reality, which is why Forrester thinks there is an ontology at work here. But as a minimal set of rules or procedures, justice 'has nothing to do with aiming at just goals or attempting to bring about a just situation' (cit. in Forrester 1997, p. 145).[3] In the Great Society Hayek imagined, justice is minimised to individuals and families seeking their own private goods, again chiefly in the market. Meanwhile, questions of human purpose are relegated to the private realm. Procedural justice has no common good, shared goals or neighbourliness in view. Indeed, for Hayek such terms smack of the stifling, not least moral collectivism, the 'teleocracy' (cit. in Forrester p. 150) he discerned in fascist and socialist totalitarianisms. Rather than heeding a just order, 'interpersonal transactions are a "game" in which the behaviour of the players, but not the result, can be just or unjust, and the behaviour includes the intentions of the players'. Hence it may be unjust to *intend* to damage another person or their interest, but 'justice is not concerned with those unintended consequences of a spontaneous order which have not been deliberately brought about by anybody' (p. 147).

This narrative certainly accompanies the DRGs. The problems we noted earlier are not identified as result of the intrinsic logic of a coherent political-economic agenda (which requires deliberative re-conception). Rather, they appear as a collection of 'unintended' consequences that can be fixed – not without a sense of naïve progressivism – if only all diverse 'stakeholders' were to procedurally collaborate (Cots et al. 2011; Bystrov et al. 2015; Numerof and Abrams 2016). Various forms of tinkering, so the hope, will minimise the 'unintended consequences' and 'maximise the intended consequences'. Again, even critics of DRGs repeat this interpretation.

The effect of this Hayekian understanding can be seen not only medicine. Despite – or because of – the increased focus on the individual as object of concern and subject of responsibility, responsibility for *systemic* decisions is diffused and untraceable, and that responsibility effectively evaporates in a field of impersonal forces. Attributable intentions together with systemic agency disappear, replaced by omission and oblivion. A single actor may be reactively picked out and sanctioned (individual cases of fraud in finance or medical institutions), which functions mainly as a deterrent. Yet the systemic question is muted. Representative political responsibility for marketisation is relegated to administrative re-organisation in the face of necessity, 'replacing the government of persons by the administration of things' (Engels cit. in Berlin 1998, p. 191).[4] Not least for this reason the marketisation of healthcare progressed slowly over decades, largely unaffected by party-political divisions. In Germany, for example, networks around the Bertelsmann Foundation since the early 1990s were particularly active in directly short-cutting to administrators. As Tanja Klenk (2011) noted, the de-politicisation of structural reforms was welcomed by left parties too. It allowed them to blame politically sensitive hospital closures on impersonal market mechanisms.

In contrast, as we saw, historically grown healthcare systems are *always already* the result of (implicit theologically grounded) truth commitments. Their form at the macro, meso- and micro-level both reflects and is challenged by these commitments. Understood as the field of decision and systemic responsibility, history is the opposite of the amoral luck of 'winners' and 'losers' in the anonymity of marketised public administration. Hence the DRGs, like other 'structural reforms' must be re-included in cultural, philosophical and political negotiations. Not because they have been excluded, but because they are *already* part of them (cp. Bode and Vogd 2016).

3. The representation of care – codification and distortion

Health-economic discipline and efficiency demand the translation of medical work into quantifiable units, especially in hospitals. And by grouping 'an almost infinite number of patients receiving in patient care into a finite number of groups of comparable patients', it became possible to 'characterise more precisely the "output" of hospitals – besides "cases" – and to represent it internally and externally transparently in a way that allows for comparison between hospitals and periods' (Busse et al. 2013, p. 57). DRGs, and similarly QALYs and DALYs (Quality- or Disability-Adjusted Life Years) in England, thus suggest representation of care through repetitive identification ('A QALY is a QALY is a QALY') and codification with a distinct utilitarian drift.

Once connected to marketisation (budget projection, revenue and profit creation, competition between hospitals), this codification frequently distorts rather represents care as it is actually given:

> The system today rewards complications more than it rewards treatment without complications; it creates diagnoses instead of representing them by setting incentives that promise plenty of income. The system deters expensive treatments if they cannot or cannot adequately be coded.
>
> (Baehr 2014)

Similarly, Bartholomeyczick (2010 cit. in Bode 2016, p. 212) criticises the 'invisibility of care in the systematics of DRG-based hospital financing', where actual differences between patients' concrete needs cannot be taken into account. And because the main diagnosis is the key economically, doctors 'must only look at the diagnosis; why the patient is here, and everything else besides, plays no role. And so the patient is treated like a disease, unfortunately, not as a person' (Braun et al. 2009, cit. in Maio 2014, p. 32).

As part of the transvaluation mentioned above marketisation has created what one might call an aporetic, 'unhappy' simultaneity of total representation and non-representation. On the one hand, ever more "transparency" suggests increased measurement and control. On the other hand, this coincides with a kind of *utopianisation*: the increased non-representation of real care. It remains a 'black box' (Bode and Vogd 2016), even if not *necessarily* to the detriment of patients. For a long time, this problem was tacitly acknowledged as mental health was exempt from the DRGsystem. In this area, 'success' is particularly unpredictable and untranslatable. Even if diagnoses are identical, the length of hospitalisation depends on the doctor, the psychiatric institution, on patients themselves and their personal circumstances (Meyera and Holzer 2015; Pfister Lipp 2014).

Theologically, the situation describes the nature and possibility of images. In the Old Testament (OT), the well-known injunctions against images of God (Ex 20:4; Dtn 4:16) deny the possibility of an 'object'. God – who is who he is (Ex 3:14) – is exempt from all representation. He is a 'black box' too, who only reveals himself in words. There are images, e.g. outside the Jerusalem temple, but they are restricted to human and other creaturely forms. The main point of the injunction was to avoid the conflation of object and divinity (i.e. magic). But already in the OT this is somewhat "upset" by the idea that human beings are made in the 'image of God.' *Their* adequate representation consists in treating them with justice and mercy, especially the weakest. In the New Testament, however, with the Incarnation the divine unseen becomes seen and manifest in word, image and body. The non-representable has been represented in Christ. Conversely, Christ 're – presents' humanity to God. The human being is now partly already participating in divine plenitude – and, in turn, *its* non-representability.

What follows from this for human representations or images of the divine has generated controversy. Broadly speaking, for Eastern interpreters, images of e.g. Christ function as an index that points towards the divine; they are iconic, both hand-made paintings and divine. In Western churches, representing the un-representable results in 'profane' art as the hand-made suggestion of the plenitudinous. Art then becomes also indicative for other forms of representation – political, administrative, economic – which concern what cannot be fully captured even in the human. These areas of social life must be re-thought from and towards the non-representable, yet again without conflation (as in "politics as art"). By the same token, any reductionism is 'iconoclastic' once it comprehensively blots out its own object, the human being. And it becomes 'idolatrous' once it mistakes the image (or 'code') for the thing itself – as seen in the DRG system.

More often than not, health economists and policy-makers are well aware that DRGs, QALYs and DALYs are not the whole picture, and that every patient is different. The point of economic vehicles of calculation was never a true knowledge of the object, Vogd (2016) points out. Nonetheless, some have sought to address the gap between care and calculus by introducing 'quality measures' into the DRGs (cp. OECD 2017). But effectively this exacerbates the problem. To quantify quality means to accept the Wittgensteinian dictum that 'there is nothing beyond the text', that compassion and mutual recognition could be measured, converted and cashed in on. It 'delegitimises the non-measurable' (Maio 2014, p. 80) more emphatically. Hence, insisting that there *is* something non-representable that escapes the current system remains preferable to expanding that system: 'Every feedback and learning loop of the DRG system will only lead to a more complex representation, which prompts new adjusting movements on the provider side with the aim to even better exploit the DRG system' (Vogd 2016, p. 291).

An alternative, more 'representative' coding system would have to participatively *follow* and *respond to* actual healthcare, that which cannot be 'coded', in a way that assures its continued possibility. Every representation of an act must be a response that allows for a renewed instantiation of the act (Williams 2014, p. 67). In other words, *retrospective* systems are more adequate, and as mentioned, continue to exist alongside prospective systems. Retrospective representation in that sense is more 'iconic': a constant process of adjustment between clinical and managerial logics (and staff), albeit under the umbrella of communal, regional and national common goods (*pace* Albach et al. 2016). Consequently, health-economic considerations, financing systems and management systems need to be short-circuited with hard questions about justice for every polity, which includes hospital ownership, anti-fraud mechanisms, waste, etc. This collides with the 'market'-claim that justice consists in every individual getting what they want at any point in time, a promise transported by the 'ethical' formulas of 'patient-centredness' and 'money follows the patient' (cp. Epstein in this volume). These imply that all allocative decisions are ultimately based on arbitrary 'lines in the sand' and suggest justice presupposes wealth – which is to put the cart before the horse and hence, defer it indefinitely.[5]

4. Economic logic and vocation

The final point then, frequently made in connection with the DRGs, concerns the responsibilities of those working *within* the marketised healthcare system. As healthcare has been relocated and redefined in market terms, those interacting with patients remain standing and working at the borderline between the market system's logic and their actual responsibilities towards patients. Giovanni Maio (2014) recently described the 'overgrowth of medicine by economics' in the clinical setting by what he calls 'structural patronising'. He observes a

> mental appropriation of doctors, as they are subtly introduced to the idea of distancing themselves from their own ideals. Or at least they are implicitly taught that those are at least as important as the economic demands of the business. The danger here is that this new hierarchy of values is not explicitly mandated, but rather that doctors are subliminally guided to internalise this hierarchy, now presented as an objective necessity, so that in the end it looks like a *voluntary acceptance*.
>
> (Maio 2014, p. 29)

That includes the internalisation of time pressures, which leads to self-exploitation (burn-out) and the individual, moral internalisation of what are, in reality, structural deficits. Hence, healthcare workers have a permanently bad conscience about their putative failures. (Maio 2014, pp. 55, 86)

Maio also describes the different ways in which the 'medical logic is turned onto its head' by economic considerations: over- and under-diagnosis go hand in hand, the patient as a whole person falls out of sight; there is a lack of time and engagement as patience, conscientiousness and exchanges with colleagues are devalued under the 'dictat of time efficiency' (Maio 2014, p. 53). Indifference is legitimised.

> Now there is no longer a standardisation that puts together symptoms as one clinical picture, but a standardisation according to a purely industrial credo. Standardisation is no longer done in order to understand what is general in the particular personal history of a patient and how it can be treated effectively according to general rules and laws, but rather standardisation in order to go into a serial production with patients, and to achieve an industrial increase of efficiency. [. . .] now humans, like objects, are subjected to an industrial production process.
>
> (Maio 2014, p. 63)

Maio sees the subsequent 'moral dissonance' as going to the substance of the profession: 'As doctors are more and more deprived of their spaces of free decision and hence the possibility to identify with their profession, patients are also indirectly deprived, because they can only be well cared for if doctors practice their profession out of a deep commitment and with joy' (Maio 2014, p. 84). This clash for professionals between the economic and medical logics, ranging from subtle to stark, has been observed since the early days of DRGs (Flintrop 2006, Braun 2010). Bode (2010, p. 203) notes the system imposes a 'double reality', so that professionals have to '"serve two masters"' (Bode 2016, p. 255).

This clash of logics also has a theological dimension. It crystallises the relationship between work and enjoyment, between law and gospel. Martin Hengel (2008) has traced the notion of work as it developed in early Christianity before the backdrop of the OT and aristocratic Greco-Roman environment. The latter despised work altogether in favour of *theoría*. Although still done joyfully in paradise (a point Luther for some time underplayed), work becomes a chore after the Fall: 'Cursed is the ground because of you; in toil you shall eat of it all the days of your life' (Gen 3:17; Hengel 2008, p. 465). But this is not unambiguous. At least fruitful work is praised as a divine gift, and frequently blessings are sought for it (Qoh 3:9–12; Ps 90, 128:2). A moral duty to work is a later rabbinic development, but there's a duty not to be idle. At the same time, work is interrupted by the Sabbath for all of creation 'to participate in God's rest' (Hengel 2008, p. 437). In the NT, work is then altogether *transvalued*: Jesus' proclamation of the divine kingdom is a 'great and final "interruption"' (Hengel 2008, p. 442). Work has a double meaning now: it is a service for the divine kingdom[6] and done selflessly for the neighbour in need. The daily job for a living (Paul was a tent-maker) takes the back seat. It shouldn't be dropped though, as some of Paul's enthusiastic audiences thought.

Yet details matter in how these pairs of work and rest, and then work and worship, are interpreted. Karl Barth, for example, not only contrasted the 'idolisation' of modern industrialised work with Sabbath rest, but thought all work finds meaning in the Sabbath: 'it points [man] away from everything that he himself can will and achieve and back to what God is for him and will do for him' (cit. in Hughes 2007). The late John Hughes critiqued this Barthian differentiation between the 'active life' of worship-in-*diakonía* and employment-work as overly stark, even though that prevents the 'glib liberal celebration of capitalism and its work-ethic' (Hughes 2007, p. 15).

Esther Reed somewhat counters Barth by insisting on the redemption of work. In her view, proclaiming the hoped-for future of transfiguration and eternal resurrection, Christians are freed from the ultimacy of everyday work. Reed also insists that the resurrection means work has eternal significance because nothing included in God's future will be lost. (Reed 2010, pp. 100–104). Nonetheless, her heavy-heavenly significance of honesty, good quality work, 'respect for clients' lacks transformative implications. Especially in hospitals where a clash of the standardised-industrialised logic with the medical logic is not without victims, Reed's curious insistence on the presence of God even 'in the darkest and most cruel workplaces' seems to bridge the Barthian gap less effectively than expected. This is similar to Maio (2014), it should be added, who suggests a 'dialogue' between the economic and medical – after he has shown that the premises for such a dialogue are no longer given.

Hughes, for his part, combines the critiques of the Frankfurt School with Romantic and Catholic strands of thought. He also notes that 'labour whose only end is efficiency and functionality, free of responsibility, intellect and delight, is *sub-human* work'. Unlike the Frankfurt School's hope in the negative power of critique, however, he suggests work depends on a vision of true labour, i.e. the creative work of God. The artist is his best analogy:

> God creates purely for the sake of the thing being created, gratuitously, out of sheer delight. He does not create out of any need or lack in himself, nor instrumentally for any other purpose. God works for no other reward than his love for the thing made.
>
> (Hughes 2007, p. 226)

Hughes then thinks human work should be analogical participation in that divine labour, a 'liturgical offering to God', and hence indistinguishable from the contemplation of God.

Hughes thus somewhat drops the notion of vocation, which in the Protestant tradition recognises even the most profane work as a service to God, indeed quite so whilst remaining 'profane'. He thinks it over-exalts mere employment and under-rates the creative, beautiful aspects of work as *vita activa*. Keeping in mind the dangers that come with such a notion of vocation, however, it retains two important aspects. First, vocation is the form and being of human freedom that cannot be exhaustively explained or justified (e.g. "Why do you want to be a doctor?"). Economic expertise can also function as a service – and vocation – to this end. Second, precisely because of its correlation with freedom, vocation has a transformative potential. Care depends on a notion of freedom that transcends different immanent logics as such, as Hughes is aware. Again, the genuinely political form can hardly be subtracted, since corporate solidarity, justice and power in healthcare is *eo ipso* structural. Hence, more than a 'dialogue' between medicine and economics in Maio's sense is needed. A substantial rethinking of marketisation as a comprehensive intellectual paradigm entails relocating the political-economic in the service of medicine as an irreducible practice of solidarity-in-suffering. This implies both rethinking the economic order, and flanking critiques such as Maio's or Hughes' with political and managerial responsibilities for healthcare workers.

5. Conclusion

Theology, says Paul Ricoeur, emerges at the intersection between 'a space of experience' and 'a horizon of hope' (cit. in Gutierrez 2009, p. 323). In this sense, marketisation of healthcare is brittle in terms of its conceptualisation and invites sharp critique. Such critique is always already taking place on the theological territory briefly mapped out here.

Marketisation, exemplified by the DRG discourse, re-defines healthcare and covers up this redefinition. This transvaluation can be demasked as historically and theologically conditioned; its grounds are up for scrutiny. As shown in the first section, systematic theology provides not least a key critical heuristic for this challenge, the opposition between political economy and the notion of care and healing. The welfare state as one specific mediate institution between medicine and market is an occasion at which this theological mediation moves into institutional forms. In concrete cases, this can lead to state-bureaucratic and managerial distortions as well as different kinds of complicities. Equally, non-state forms of care provision such as social entrepreneurship and diaconic organisations can function as such mediate institutions.

With reference to Hayek, we have also seen how the market paradigm generates ahistoricity as well as a lack of political responsibility (and imagination), exemplified in the way DRGs were implemented. Against this I have emphasised both the significance of history for any institution to be legitimate; and for marketisation to be re-embedded into political responsibilities, not least grounded in the interpretations of the past.

The problem of representation through coding systems such as the DRG was raised: they distort and re-direct care away from its *sui generis* task. An adequate representation of care, however, has to be truthful in that it neither distorts nor blots out its own object, but rather furthers its continued re-instantiation. This connected to the final point: problematic contradictions *within* the profession created by marketisation, which will also be dealt with in more detail in Part III of this volume. Here different theological approaches find ways to conceptualise and resolve the present fissure between the economic and medical logic. Granular differences matter; Protestant/Reformed emphases on vocation eschatologically shift perspectives, or transformatively re-orient structures; the Catholic emphasis, more integral, emphasises dialogue and a creative-artisan fulfillment of work.

For all their differences, these approaches imply that healthcare's corporate-personal responsibility cannot be absorbed into a jargon of 'hybridisation' or 'balancing' contradictory tensions within a grid of maximising personal utility. Marketisation is not complete, as an intellectual paradigm, a jargon or a practice. The various critiques over the years have shown that a continuous exercise of freedom, politics, creativity and care *can* reverse the transvaluation of healthcare, and reorient it towards its genuine end.

Notes

1 Therese Feiler gratefully acknowledges the support from the University of Oxford Wellcome Trust Institutional Strategic Support Fund (105605/Z/14/Z) and the Arts and Humanities Research Council (AH/N009770/1).
2 Pfister Lipp (2014, pp. 59–64) identifies four areas of concern: justice of care provision, quality of care, vocational ethos and work conditions.
3 Hayek's parallels with Rawls explains their simultaneous success in the late twentieth century.
4 The irony of this twist – that marketisation engenders systems comparable to Soviet administration – should not be lost on the reader (see also Bevan and Hood 2006).
5 See Margaret Thatcher's infamous quip that the Good Samaritan needed money to pay for the victim's care. This obvious point becomes problematic if she meant to say: *first* he needed to make money, *then* he could help.
6 Mk 1:17 "Follow me, and I will make you fish for people."; Matt 9:37f; Lk 10:2. Matt 10:7–8 "As you go, proclaim the good news, 'The kingdom of heaven has come near.' Cure the sick, raise the dead, cleanse the lepers, cast out demons. You received without payment; give without payment" Cp. 1 Cor 3:9.

References

Albach, H. et al. (eds.) (2016) *Boundaryless Hospital: Rethink and Redefine Health Care Management.* Heidelberg, Berlin: Springer.

Baehr, M. (2014) Fallpauschalen: Schweden setzt richtige Anreize. *Deutsches Ärzteblatt*, 111 (46), A-2003/B-1713/C-1639. [Online] Available from: www.aerzteblatt.de/archiv/163583 [Accessed 18 July 2017]

Balleisen, E. J. (2017) *Fraud: An American History from Barnum to Madoff.* Princeton, Oxford: Princeton University Press.

Bell, Jr., D. M. (2005) Only Jesus Saves: Toward a Theopolitical Ontology of Judgment. In: Davis, C., Milbank, J., and Žižek, S. (eds.) *Theology and the Political: The New Debate.* Durham, London: Duke University Press, pp. 200–228.

Benjamin, W. (1991) Kapitalismus als Religion [Fragment]. In: Tiedemann, R., Schweppenhäuser, H., and Benjamin, W. (eds.) *Gesammelte Schriften.* Frankfurt am Main: Suhrkamp, vol. 6, pp. 100–102.

Berlin, I. (1998) *The Proper Study of Mankind: An Anthology of Essays.* London: Pimlico.

Bevan, G., and Hood, C. (2006) What's Measured Is What Matters: Targets and Gaming in the English Public Health Care System. *Public Administration*, 84 (3), 517–538.

Bode, I. (2010), Die Malaise der Krankenhäuser, *Leviathan*, 38, 189–211.

Bode, I. (2011) The Re-Organization of Inpatient Care in Germany: Competing institutional logics and hybrid accountability. EON-Ruhrgas Scholarship Conference: *The Changing Organization of the Welfare State – Between Efficiency and Accountability*, Potsdam.

Bode, I. (2016) Stress durch rekursive Ambivalenz: Oder: Wie und warum das Krankenhauswesen mutiert. In: Bode, I. and Vogd, W. (eds.) *Mutationen des Krankenhauses: Soziologische Diagnosen in organisations- und gesellschaftstheoretischer Perspektive.* Wiesbaden: Springer, pp. 253–280.

Bode, I., and Vogd, W. (2016) Einleitung. In: Bode, I. and Vogd, W. (eds.) *Mutationen des Krankenhauses: Soziologische Diagnosen in organisations- und gesellschaftstheoretischer Perspektive.* Wiesbaden: Springer, pp. 1–28.

Bonhoeffer, D. (2009) *Works, Vol. 6: Ethics.* Minneapolis, MN: Fortress Press.

Braun, B. (2014) Auswirkungen der DRGs auf Versorgungsqualität und Arbeitsbedingungen im Krankenhaus. In: Manzei, A., and Schmiede, R. (eds.) *20 Jahre Wettbewerb im Gesundheitswesen: Theoretische und empirische Analysen zur Ökonomisierung von Medizin und Pflege.* Wiesbaden: Springer, pp. 91–113.

Braun, B., Klinke, S., and Müller, R. (2010) Auswirkungen des DRG-Systems auf die Arbeitssituation im Pflegebereich von Akutkrankenhäusern. *Pflege & Gesellschaft*, 15 (1), 5–19.

Brennan, L. et al. (2012) The Importance of Knowing Context of Hospital Episode Statistics When Reconfiguring the NHS. *BMJ*, 344, e2432.

Burke, S. A. et al. (2016) From Universal Health Insurance to Universal Healthcare? The Shifting Health Policy Landscape in Ireland since the Economic Crisis. *Health Policy*, 120 (3), 235–240.

Busse, R., Tiemann, O., and Schreyögg, J. (2013) Leistungsmanagement in Krankenhäusern. In: Busse, R., Schreyögg, J., and Stargardt, T. (eds.) *Management im Gesundheitswesen: Das Lehrbuch für Studium und Praxis.* Berlin, Heidelberg: Springer, pp. 51–76.

Bystrov, V. et al. (2015) Effects of DRG-Based Hospital Payment in Poland on Treatment of Patients with Stroke. *Health Policy*, 119 (8), 1119–1125.

Chambers, S., Arora, M., and Arora, A. (2010) Payment by Results and Elderly Care Medicine – Friend or Foe? *GM Journal*, 40, Oct., 529–539.

Chilingerian, J. (2008) Origins of DRGs in the United States: A Technical, Political and Cultural Story. In: John Kimberly, J., Gerard de Pouvourville, G., and Thomas d'Aunno, T. (eds.) *The Globalization of Managerial Innovation in Health Care*. Cambridge: Cambridge University Press, pp. 4–33

Cooper, C. (2016) Pressure on Hospitals to 'Cook the Books'. *The Independent*, Feb. 16. [Online] Available from: www.independent.co.uk/news/pressure-on-hospitals-to-cook-the-books

Cots, F. et al. (2011) DRG-Based Hospital Payment: Intended and Unintended Consequences. In: Busse, R. et al. (eds.) *Diagnosis-Related Groups in Europe: Moving towards Transparency, Efficiency and Quality in Hospitals*. Maidenhead: McGraw Hill Open University Press, pp. 75–92.

Department of Health. (2013) *Payment by Results in the NHS: A Simple Guide*. [Online] Available from: www.gov.uk/government/uploads/system/uploads/attachment_data/file/213150/PbR-Simple-Guide-FINAL.pdf [Accessed 18 July 2017]

Flintrop, J. (2006) Auswirkungen der DRG-Einführung: Die ökonomische Logik wird zum Maß der Dinge. *Deutsches Ärzteblatt*, 103 (46), A-3082/B-2683 /C-2574.

Forrester, D. B. (1997) *Christian Justice and Public Policy*. Cambridge: Cambridge University Press.

Frey, J., Krauter, S., and Lichtenberger, H. (2009) Einleitung, In: Frey, J., Krauter, S., and Lichtenberger, H. (eds.) *Heil und Geschichte: Die Geschichtsbezogenheit des Heils und das Problem der Heilsgeschichte in der biblischen Tradition und in der theologischen Deutung*. Tübingen: Mohr Siebeck, pp. XI-XXX.

Gaffney, A. (2014) The Neoliberal Turn in American Health Care: The Failings of the Affordable Care Act Are Rooted in a Long Shift Away from the Idea of a Truly Universal Health Care. *The Jacobin*, Apr. 15, 2014 [Online] Available from: www.jacobinmag.com/2014/04/the-neoliberal-turn-in-american-health-care/ [Accessed 2 June 2016]

Gutierrez, G. (2009) The Option for the Poor Arises from Faith in Christ. *Theological Studies*, 70 (2), 317–326.

Hayek, F. A. v. (1982) *Law, Legislation and Liberty*, vol. I: *Rules and Order*. London: Routledge and Paul Kegan.

Hengel, M. (2008) *Studien zum Urchristentum. Kleine Schriften VI*. Tübingen: Mohr-Siebeck.

Hughes, J. (2007) *The End of Work: Theological Critiques of Capitalism*. Oxford: Blackwell.

Kidwell, J., and Doherty, S. (eds.) (2015) *Theology and Economics: A Christian Vision of the Common Good*. New York: Palgrave Macmillan.

Kimberly, J., Pouvourville, G. D., and D'Aunno, T. (eds.) (2008) *The Globalization of Managerial Innovation in Health Care*. Cambridge: Cambridge University Press.

Klenk, T. (2011) Ownership Change and the Rise of a For-Profit Hospital Industry in Germany. *Policy Studies*, 32 (3), 263–275.

Long, D. S., Fox, N. R., and York, T. (2007) *Calculated Futures: Theology, Ethics, and Economics*. Waco, TX: Baylor University Press.

Maio, G. (2014) *Geschäftsmodell Gesundheit: Wie der Markt die Heilkunst abschafft*. Berlin: Suhrkamp.

Marshall, L., Charlesworth, A., and Hurst, J. (2014) *The NHS Payment System: Evolving Policy and Emerging Evidence*. [Online] Available from: www.nuffieldtrust.org.uk/research/the-nhs-payment-system-evolving-policy-and-emerging-evidence [Accessed 18 July, 2017]

Mathauer, I., and Wittenbecher, F. (2013) Hospital Payment Systems Based on Diagnosis-Related Groups: Experiences in Low- and Middle-Income Countries. *Bulletin of the World Health Organization*, 91, 746–756A.

Meyera, B., and Holzer, B. (2015) Leistungsbezogenes Tarifsystem für die stationäre Psychiatrie Schweizerische Ärztezeitung. *Bulletin Des Médecins Suisses/Bollettino Dei Medici Svizzeri*, 96 (25), 902–904.

Milbank, J. (2015) The Moral Limits of Markets. In: Skidelsky, E., and Skidelsky, R. (eds.) *Are Markets Moral? (Symposium) (2013: London, England)*. Basingstoke, Hampshire: Palgrave Macmillan, pp. 77–102.

Neby, S. et al. (2015) Bending the Rules to Play the Game Accountability, DRG and Waiting List Scandals in Norway and Germany. *European Policy Analysis*, 1 (1), 127–148.

Numerof, R. E., and Abrams, M. (2016) *Bringing Value to Healthcare: Practical Steps for Getting to a Market-Based Model*. Boca Raton, FL: CRC, Productivity Press.

OECD Health Project. (2004) *Towards High-Performing Health Systems*. Paris: OECD Publishing.

OECD High Level Reflection Group on the Future of Health Statistics. (2017) *Recommendations to OECD Ministers of Health: Strengthening the International Comparison of Health System Performance through Patient-Reported Indicators*. Paris: OECD Publishing.

Patzen, M. (2010) Qualität und Ethik in Gefahr durch DRG? *Competence*, 5, 31.

Petratos, P. (2018) Why the Economic Calculation Debate Matters: The Case for Decentralisation in Healthcare. In: Feiler, T., Hordern, J., and Papanikitas, A. (eds.) *Marketisation, Ethics and Healthcare: Policy, Practice and Moral Formation*. Abingdon: Routledge, pp. 13–31.

Pfister Lipp, E. (2014) *Die Rolle der Ethik in der Gesundheitspolitik: Eine philosophisch-empirische Untersuchung anhand der DRG-Reform in der Schweiz*. Berlin: LIT Verlag.

Ramsey, P. (2016) *Speak Up for Just War or Pacifism*. 2nd ed. Eugene, OR: Wipf and Stock.

Reed, E. D. (2010) *Work, for God's Sake: Christian Ethics in the Workplace*. London: Darton, Longman and Todd.

Savulescu, J., and Schuklenk, U. (2017) Doctors Have no Right to Refuse Medical Assistance in Dying, Abortion or Contraception. *Bioethics*, 31 (3), 162–170.

Schaper, J. (2009) "Dann sollst du anheben und sagen vor dem Herrn, deinem Gott . . . ": Heil, Geschichte und Gedächtnis im Deuteronomium. In: Frey, J., Krauter, S., and Lichtenberger, H. (eds.) *Heil und Geschichte: die Geschichtsbezogenheit des Heils und das Problem der Heilsgeschichte in der biblischen Tradition und in der theologischen Deutung*. Tübingen: Mohr Siebeck, pp. 65–73.

Skidelsky, E., and Skidelsky, R. (eds.) *Are Markets Moral?* (Symposium) (2013: London, England). Basingstoke, Hampshire: Palgrave Macmillan

Turre, R. (1991) *Diakonik: Grundlegung und Gestaltung der Diakonie*. Neukirchen-Vluyn: Neukirchener.

Vogd, W. (2016) Das Missverstehen des Ökonomischen: Oder vom Sündenfall falsch verstandener Rationalitäten im Krankenhaus. In: Bode, I. and Vogd, W. (eds.) *Mutationen des Krankenhauses: Soziologische Diagnosen in organisations- und gesellschaftstheoretischer Perspektive*. Wiesbaden: Springer, pp. 281–308.Wegner, G. (2015) Einleitung. In: Wegner, G. (ed.) *Die Legitimität des Sozialstaates: Religion – Gender – Neoliberalismus*. Leipzig: Evangelische Verlagsanstalt, pp. 7–26.

Williams, R. (2014) *The Edge of Words: God and the Habits of Language*. London: Bloomsbury.

Zimmermann-Acklin, M. (2010) *Bioethik in theologischer Perspektive: Grundlagen, Methoden, Bereiche*. 2nd ed. Freiburg, Vienna: Herder.

5 Personal budgets

Holding onto the purse strings for fear of something worse

Jonathan Herring

Introduction

The past decade has witnessed a dramatic shift in the approach of the state towards social care. We are now in an era of personalisation and individual budgets (Department of Health 2007; Clements 2008; Poole 2007). Rather than the local authority providing services and equipment to meet someone's care needs, the person in need is given a budget that they can use to purchase the services they require. These may be purchased from the local authority or other providers. The aim is to put people in charge of determining how to meet their care needs. The Department of Health (2010: 15) set out its vision:

> Our vision starts with securing the best outcomes for people. People, not service providers or systems, should hold the choice and control about their care. Personal budgets and direct payments are a powerful way to give people control. Care is a uniquely personal service. It supports people at their most vulnerable, and often covers the most intimate and private aspects of their lives. With choice and control, people's dignity and freedom is protected and their quality of life is enhanced. Our vision is to make sure everyone can get the personalised support they deserve.

So expressed, it might seem surprising that anyone would object to such approach. However, in this chapter I will be largely critical of these developments.

Much has been written based on empirical studies about the effectiveness of the use of personal budgets. It is too early to be able to form a definitive view on that. The Social Care Institute for Excellence (2011: 2), in their review, found that:

> Evaluations so far indicate that PBs have resulted in marginally improved outcomes across a across a range of different groups. There is a degree of variation among these groups though: people with learning disabilities and mental health conditions have shown the most improvement (though those with mental health conditions are least likely to be offered a PB), while older people have reported the lowest level of improvement in outcomes; in one or two areas they have seen a negative drop in outcomes when compared with control groups.

In this chapter, I will be exploring the issue from a more theoretical perspective. I regard personal budgets as an expression of consumerist personal autonomy. In order to be effective, consumerism relies on the market responding to improve quality and reduced costs. I will argue that a reliance on consumerism in this instance is based on a false view of autonomy and fails to adequately appreciate the nature of care.

The personalised care provision, centred around personal budgets, offers a market based response which intends to enable people to live independent, empowered, self-determined lives. However, that is an offer which should be rejected. Good care is not about independence but interdependence. Good care is not about empowering, but sharing our vulnerabilities. Good care is not about self-determination, but a mutual sharing of our relational autonomies. Care cannot be packaged, valued, or budgeted. In its nature it is relational, involving responsibilities and intermingling of interests and identities. Care is something we all do and we all need. It is not placing a burden on others; it is being human. Our social interventions need to rejoice in care and enable and support it. Presenting it as a marketised package is wrong starting point.

Before expanding on that critique, I will start by summarising the legal framework for personal budgets.

1. Care Act 2014 and personal budgets

Personal budgets in England date back to the Community Care (Direct Payments) Act of 1996, which empowered local authorities to give cash payments to service users in place of direct services. In 2001 the Government issued guidance that required Local Authority social services departments to offer certain people direct cash payments to spend on discrete items of care and support. These were gradually developed to become personal budgets and become used throughout social care (Department of Health 2007).

The Care Act 2014, for the first time, put personal budgets on a statutory footing. In the Government White Paper, the Government (2012: 19) promised through the legislation to extend the use of personal budgets, saying:

> We will transform people's experience of care and support, putting them in control and ensuring that services respond to what they want. We will ensure that people have control over their budget and their care and support plan, and will empower them to choose and to shape the options that best enable them to meet their goals and aspirations.

Under the 2014 Act, the local authority will assess the care needs of a person. This should be done in consultation with the person needing care: "This process will decide how to meet the needs of the person, and the local authority must do everything it reasonably can to reach agreement with the person as to how their needs should be met" (Department of Health 2011: 1). Personal budgets are one way that can be used as an appropriate way to meet their care needs. While it is not compulsory to use a personal budget, they are "the Government's preferred mechanism for personalised care and support" (Department of Health 2014: para 12.2). They are intended to become "the norm for people with care and support needs" (Department of Health 2014: para 11.2). However, significantly, the Care Act makes it clear they can only be used where someone requests them. The statutory guidance states: "People must not be forced to take a direct payment against their will, but instead be informed of the choices available to them" (Department of Health 2014: para 12.5).

Section 31 of the Care Act 2014 states that adults with capacity[1] who have care needs can request direct payment as a personal budget and the local authority must comply with this, if four conditions are met:

(4)   Condition 1 is that –

the adult has capacity to make the request, and
where there is a nominated person, that person agrees to receive the payments.

(5)   Condition 2 is that –

the local authority is not prohibited by regulations under section 33 from meeting the adult's needs by making direct payments to the adult or nominated person, and
if regulations under that section give the local authority discretion to decide not to meet the adult's needs by making direct payments to the adult or nominated person, it does not exercise that discretion.

(6)   Condition 3 is that the local authority is satisfied that the adult or nominated person is capable of managing direct payments –

by himself or herself, or
with whatever help the authority thinks the adult or nominated person will be able to access.

(7)   Condition 4 is that the local authority is satisfied that making direct payments to the adult or nominated person is an appropriate way to meet the needs in question.

If the conditions are met a person has a "right" to receive direct payments. However as Belinda Schwehr (2016) points out: "since two of the conditions allow for much difference of professional judgement, on the same facts, one would never safely call it 'a right'." She has in mind the requirements three and four, where there is ample scope for a council to determine a person does not have the capability to manage the payment or that it is not appropriate to pay the money to the user. The statutory guidance (Department of Health 2011: para 12.18) states: "Where refused, the person or person making the request should be provided with written reasons that explain the decision, and be made aware of how to appeal the decision through the local complaints process."

The personal budget will give clear guidance as to how much money has been allocated to meet the identified needs. The budget will be based on the care and support plan that is drawn up with P's involvement and indeed "it should be made clear that the plan 'belongs' to the person it is intended for, with the local authority role to ensure the production and sign-off of the plan to ensure that it is appropriate to meet the identified needs" (Department of Health 2014: para 10.2). P can determine what set of services will best meet their needs; who would be the best provider of those services; and the details about when and how the services should be provided. The idea behind persona budget is that P will use them to purchase the services they need. They are put in control of their care provision (Carr and Hunter 2012). The Statutory Guidance states it will provide great choice and allow people to "take control" over how their needs are met (Department of Health 2014: para 1.2). This might include how often they receive the care (some people might, for example, prefer a smaller number of longer visits to a larger number of shorter visits); or when they receive visits (if they need care at particular times they can contract to ensure that occurs); who provides the care (they may select people know to them); or ensure care meets personal preferences (e.g. that they are provided by a religious organisation).

There are a range of ways a personal budget can be operated. They do not necessarily involve P having direct control, although in all the versions, P is meant to have a degree of control. They include the following:

- As a managed account held by the local authority with support provided in line with the person's wishes;
- As a managed account held by a third party with support provided in line with the persons wishes;
- As a direct payment.

If the budget is handed over to P or someone acting on their behalf, the council can restrict in what it can be used for.[2] In particular, the service purchased must be a service which the council could have provided. So it could certainly not be used for registered nurse nursing care or long term residential care, as a local authority could not provide these using a care budget. Belinda Schwehr (2016) lists the follow as more debatable cases:

> Help with having sex – because although buying sex is not illegal, and could be highly relevant to the development of new relationships after someone has had an accident, councils are probably entitled to a policy on spending on particular things, to protect themselves from having to deal with harm to their own reputations.
>
> Entertainment fees for an event, for a person for whom mainstream recreation is not inaccessible by reason of their particular disability or condition.
>
> Hedge funds (however profitable!), gambling (however exhilarating), alcohol, cigarettes (although neither are illegal), drugs of any sort including homeopathic remedies, and actual food for someone who has no condition-related difficulty in accessing adequate nutrition and hydration.

An important new obligation is put on the local authority through section 5 which puts a duty on local authority to take reasonable steps to achieve a vibrant, responsive market of service providers. It states:

> A local authority must promote the efficient and effective operation of a market in services for meeting care and support needs with a view to ensuring that any person in its area wishing to access services in the market –
>
> • has a variety of providers to choose from who (taken together) provide a variety of services;
> • has a variety of high quality services to choose from;
> • has sufficient information to make an informed decision about how to meet the needs in question.

Detailed guidance on how this duty should be performed has been produced by the Department of Health (2017). Sections 19 and 48–57 provide detailed guidance on the responsibilities of local authorities where there is a business failure impacting the provision of services. These provisions reflect the fact that as Kelly (2013: 74) notes, although social care is the responsibility of local authorities "few . . . are now involved in the direct delivery of care and support services", with most services operated by private providers.

2. Personalisation

A key theme in the move towards personal budgets and indeed more broadly in modern approaches to adult care (Owens, Mladenov and Cribb 2016), has been the move to personalisation (Needham 2011). This requires that the focus should be on the goals and wishes of the individual (P). P should be involved in determining what their goals are and be helped to achieve them. At first sight that seems to be a very sensible approach. Who else better to decide what is in P's best interests then P themselves? It avoids the state or another person determining how people should live their lives. As *Putting People First* puts it, 'The time has now come to build on best practice and replace *paternalistic, reactive care of variable quality* with a mainstream system focussed on prevention, early intervention, enablement and high quality personally tailored services' (Department of Health 2007: 2). The Social Care Institute of Excellence (2012: 3) explains:

> At the heart of personalisation is the commitment to giving more choice and control to people using social care services. This may mean exploring personal budget options but it could also mean working with individuals in residential settings to ensure that their personal needs and preferences are identified and met. It is about self-directed support and enabling people to make their own decisions about what care and support they require to lead a full and independent life.

The Statutory Guidance (Department of Health 2014: para 11.2) gives the kind of example which is commonly used drawn on in support of personal budgets:

> Sally really enjoys dancing and night clubs and she needs support for this. Sally's ISF [Individual Service Funds] arrangement with her provider has given her the flexibility to employ staff that also like to do this, and they are paid time and a half after 11:00pm. The ISF arrangement also allows Sally to convert 'standard hours' into 'enhanced hours', for example, 6 standard hours equals 4 enhanced hours. Sally can plan late nights out knowing what it 'costs' from her allocation of 24 standard hours support, which is calculated from her personal budget.

Personal budgets have received judicial support. In the Supreme Court in *R (KM) v Cambridgeshire* [2012] UKSC 23 Lord Wilson said of the scheme, 'The admirable idea is to empower him with control over his own budget'(para 23).

The Guidance for the Care Act of 2014 cites research it says shows that if implemented well, personal budgets can provide better care and value for money than local authority sourced services (Department of Health 2014). There seems to be some debate about that. The Audit Commission (2008) has stated it believes personal budgets will be cost-neutral and that there are not expected to be large savings. The IBSEN evaluation found "very small savings" (Glendinning et al. 2008) with personal budgets.

3. Autonomy and stress

Even if a person chooses to take on a personal budget, this can become a cause of significant distress and worry. This is particularly where a person may feel "abandoned" when making their own choices. The skill and effort needed to find and negotiate care should not be underestimated (Glendinning 2007). Ann Stewart (2005), in a powerful personal account, tells of the difficulties she faced in obtaining services for her parents. Despite having a good grasp of the legal and practical issues – being an academic specialising in the area – the commissioning and supervision of services was extremely burdensome. As she points out, others will be in a much less privileged position than she was.

The benefits of autonomy need to weighed against the stress and worry caused to P and/or their friends and relatives (Woolham et al. 2016). Indeed, one survey reported that individual budgets, far from lessening the burden on those caring for dependent relatives, had led to them having to take on the extra responsibilities of managing the personal budgets (Glendinning et al. 2009).

A good example of the stress that can arise is the use of personal budgets to employ carers. Carers UK (2011) list some of the responsibilities that a person employing a carer will need to make:

> check the references of the intended employee and find out if they have had an up to date Disclosure and Barring Service (DBS) check make sure the

intended employee has the right to work in the UK set up a system for paying wages, deducting tax and national insurance and keeping records for the
Inland Revenue ensure that the employee has the annual leave they are entitled
to under 'Working Time Regulations', any maternity/paternity/sick pay they
are entitled to and ensure you comply with auto enrolment duties do a check
to ensure that there are no potential health and safety risks to the employee
because of the care they will be providing, as well as removing any potential
dangers in your home that could put them at risk ensure that you have suitable insurance cover (i.e. employer's liability insurance and public liability
insurance).

These would be daunting for anyone, let alone a person reliant on local authority
care or their family members. This is why many people rely on care agencies to
find and employ carers, but this, inevitably, limits the control the service user has
over the delivery of care.

The management of personal budgets can involve not only the finding and management of care provision, but also the keeping of records and the submission
of accounts to the local council to show how the money was spent. Baxter and
Glendinning (2013) found personal budgets causing significant emotional costs.
As they point out, these do not necessarily outweigh the benefits of choice, but
need to be put alongside it.

4. Autonomy and carers

The traditional image of care has been one of a passive recipient of care receiving
assistance from a skilled carer. One of the reasons given to support personal budgets
is that it challenges that presentation. As Fiona Williams (2001: 468) comments:

> I would suggest that, in so far as this move to direct payments has also been,
> in part, and in some places, the consequence of demands from the disability
> movement, then it indicates not simply a 'distancing', but also a challenge to
> the assumed, all-encompassing dependency of the 'cared-for' in care relations
> and practices.

This reflects the concerns of some that the notion of care, paints a picture of the
person "receiving care" as the passive recipient of care. Personal budgets enable
them to direct the level of care and become the director of it. It responds to the
concern that:

> The concept of care seems to many disabled people a tool through which
> others are able to dominate and manage our lives.
>
> (Wood 1989: 199)

This argument is a persuasive critique of how care is sometimes portrayed. However, the response to it need not be a "personal assistant model" where by the

person receiving care directs the assistant in what they should do. I have argued elsewhere a preferable response is:

> to emphasise that we should seek to promote caring relationships, not just carers. We should emphasise that respect is central to good care, and that, most importantly, in the caring relationships we are all in there is a merging of interests and selves. Vulnerabilities, care and identities become mutual and interdependent. We need to break down the division between the 'carer' and the 'cared for', between the 'disabled' and the 'able-bodied'. Instead, we need to recognise our mutual vulnerability and need for care and ensure that there is a fair division of the burden and costs attached to caring relationships.
>
> (Herring 2014b: 2)

The use of personal budgets to create a model whereby P employs a "carer" whose job it is to enable P to be autonomous has dangers of undermining the interest of "carers", just as the traditional image of care has demeaned those who "receive care". Maketisation in this field can therefore impact on senses of identity and vocation among those involved in personal care.

It should not be thought that the Care Act of 2014 is all bad news for "carers". One important aspect of personal budgets is that it does mean that some informal carers, especially those not living with the individual, can receive pay for their care work when they would not otherwise receive that pay. Clare Ungerson (2004: 189) has argued:

> by allowing for the payment of relatives who previously have been 'classic' unpaid and formally unrecognised informal carers, [these schemes] actually provide a means whereby the work of care-givers is recognised and recompensed, such that they become more and more like care-workers.

The Act also allows "carers" to be assessed in their own right and to be given services or budgets to meet their needs.

However, as indicated there are reasons for "carers" to be nervous about the use of personal budgets. First, it is generally assumed that the scheme of personal budgets assumes there is not a clash between the between the interests of the 'carer' and the 'cared for' (Keywood 2003). The comments of one carer are the kind typically cited:

> Much as I love him, I have no interest in my husband's hobbies – now I don't have to be involved in them as his workers are. It gives him something to tell me about or if he wants can keep it private, something he hasn't had for a long time. Direct payments suit us perfectly.
>
> (Carers UK 2011: 3)

However, the assumption of a coincidence of interests does not follow. P may decide not to use their budget on receiving a service the authority previously provided and so increase the burden on the carer. The day in the day-centre visit replaced by a couple of hours fishing may well better meet the needs of P but lead to an increase in the burden on P's "carer" and contribute to the closure of the day-centre.

Second, although the Care Act 2014 does allow local authorities to asses carers (Mitchell and Glendinning 2016). This has proved problematic in practice. The major study on this to date finds a significant disparity in the way eligibility criteria are interpreted and how carers' needs are assessed (Glendinning, Mitchell and Brooks 2014). The criteria, based around the concepts of regular and substantial care, were found to be unclear and varied. One survey found only 4.8% of carer respondents had their own personal budget (Hatton and Waters 2013). I suspect this is because many carers do not see their needs as analogous to the person they are caring for. There is a further difficulty and that is that assessing "carers" and "those with needs" separately overlooks the interdependency between people and the way their identities become intertwined (Mitchell and Glendinning 2016).

Third, for people who are professional carers, there are significant concerns. The vulnerability of their position is already well known, with a series of scandals involving low paid and poor working conditions. The existence of personal budgets may simply increase the difficulties. Now these workers will be answerable not only to the companies over seeing their services, but those receiving care will have the power to control and determine services (Owens, Mladenov and Cribb 2016).

5. Autonomy and individualism

Much of the government literature promoting personal budgets has an indivdi-ualised conception of autonomy: with P determining how they want "their needs" meet. However, few us in fact make decisions in this way. We make decision in consultation with others. Not least because we realise that few of our problems are "our own", but the decisions we make will impact on others and rely on others to be successful. It is such observations which promote the concept of relational autonomy, which emphasises the importance of appreciating the relational context within which decisions need to be made and within which they can be carried out (Herring 2014a).

A relational autonomy approach would question much of the presentation of "autonomy" portrayed in the personal budget rhetoric. Indeed, one of the interest-ing things to emerge from the growth of personal budgets is formal and informal networks of support among "service users". One prominent example is the Norfolk Coalition of Disabled people, which brings together user-led groups to offer sup-port planning for people with personal budgets, to share knowledge and support. The emergence of these demonstrates that people do not want to make these deci-sions on their own.

While the growth of these informal groups is welcome, we must appreciate that not all will have the kind of relational networks of support that relational autonomy would require. The Government's personal budget literature does not seem to rec-ognise that while there are some well informed and well connected people who can draw on significant relational resources in excising autonomy, there are others who have chronic mental or physical ill health or are isolated and lack relational support (Barnes 2011). This reflects a broader point that consumerist accounts of autonomy favour those who are autonomous. It is notable that the assessment of P's needs, which plays such a key part in the process, is often carried out without involving P in a relational way. Slasberg, Beresford and Schofield (2013: 104) argue:

> The assessment process has become increasingly dominated by questionnaires with closed questions. This is not experienced as conducive to the nature of conversations that are engaging and empowering; decisions about resource allocation are being carried out by professionals where the service user is not present.

Even if P is involved, there seems to be a reluctance in some local authorities to involve their family (Hamilton et al. 2016). This ties into the issues relating to carers above. An assessment needs to be made of the caring relationships and what services are needed to support these, rather than attempting to assess the individuals separately. Rather than an assessment of P alone or without involving those in caring relationships with P.

6. Autonomy and shifting responsibility

A cynic might suggest that the use of personal budgets means that the local authority can wash its hands of responsibilities of care (Spandler 2004). If an individual is not receiving appropriate care, or the services are inadequate, the local authority cannot be blamed (Ferguson 2007). The person has simply misused their budget. It reinforces the perception that primary responsibility for care lies not with the state but with individuals, families and charities. that chimes with the themes privatisation, commoditisation and individualism (Pollock 2005). As Social Care Institute for Excellence (2011: 3) acknowledges:"[Personalisation] is not a value neutral term, and can be used to signal a variety of different policy intentions, from transferring risk and responsibility away from the state, to a new model of social citizenship".

The use of personal budgets at a time of "austerity" creates particular fears that they can be ready vehicles for masking cuts in social care spending (Owens, Mladenov and Cribb 2016). In particular, there is risk with increased political discussion that individuals should be expected to save for, or insure against, future care needs, that we are seeing the withdrawal of state funding of care.

7. Autonomy and reality of choice

While autonomy can be said to promote choice and freedom, it is important to appreciate that choice is not always experienced in this way. While it is clear in the Care Act that the person must choose to seek a personal budget, there is also in the accompanying literature a strong push for personal budgets to be the norm. The message that a person will be disempowered if they do not agree to personal budgets is a powerful one and is likely to lead people to feel pressured to accept a budget, especially if they expected it and were encouraged to do so by professionals (Owens, Mladenov and Cribb 2016). A survey for Carers UK (2011: 2) found 5% of those surveyed said they had been pressured into accepting direct payments.

Even if having a personal budget is freely chosen, the range of choices available for the provision of services may be limited. There may be few providers who are available, particularly within the costs permitted within the local authority budget. In particular, there is a concern that "the personalisation agenda has often been accompanied by the introduction of measures that seek to bring service users' decisions into line with the agendas of policy-makers and services providers" (Owens, Mladenov and Cribb 2016). These concerns are particularly acute, as a service user often has more limited material, social, economic, political and personal resources with which to explore options and may be very dependent on the local authority for assistance in exercising their choice. Autonomy, in other words is not just a matter of giving a person a choice, but ensuring there is in place broad social and person conditions within which a person can exercise a meaningful choice. The negative assumptions about "welfare recipients", ageist attitudes, and depression amongst older people can all work to limit and impact on choice. Morris (2003) also highlights the difficulties in finding services:

> People who use direct payments consistently report difficulties in recruiting personal assistants. Poor rates of pay create situations where disabled people are forced to take on personal assistants who cannot provide them with a good service. If support needs are not properly funded, personal assistance service users find they cannot provide good working conditions for their workers.

In such an environment, talk of choice may ring a little hollow.

Further, for P to make an autonomous choice they must have capacity and that involves having an understanding of the key facts and a choice between two options. One concern is that common for people to hide from their weakness and be overly optimistic. Is P really in a position to understand their own state. Are they able to properly assess the market for care services and know which provider to select? (Glasby and Beresford 2006) Have they come to terms with their current condition or are they still working it through? Notably in one study of 600 social workers 96% were concerned that service users would be more vulnerable if personal budgets were extended (Mickel 2008). Only 11% thought it appropriate to extend personal budgets to all users. Indeed, it is notable that many service users rely on a third party to control their budgets. For example, Direct Payments Service Users Ltd was set up in Nottinghamshire and ran the accounts of over 3000 people care needs. However, with such large scale operations, one wonders whether the language of autonomy and personalisation are misplaced (Glendinning 2008).

8. Autonomy and abuse

A particular concern is that a personal budget holder may be open to financial abuse (Manthorpe and Samsi 2013). The problem of financial abuse of older people is well recorded and notoriously difficult to identify and harder still to prosecute (Collins 2014). There is evidence of personal budgets being targeted by fraudsters (e.g. *R (G & H) v North Somerset Council* [2011] EWHC 2232 (Admin)). In *R (Collins) v Nottinghamshire County Council* [2016] EWHC 996 (Admin), the court addressed a case involving Direct Payments Services Users Ltd whose accreditation was removed by the council after serious financial allegations were discovered involving fraudulent use of services users accounts. Ismail et al. (2017) found evidence of much smaller scale fraud with home care employees engaging in financial abuse of those with personal budgets.

9. Concluding thoughts

Underpinning many of the concerns expressed in this chapter is that personal budgets and marketisation fail to appreciate the true nature of care (Leece 2004). It is not recognised for being something that is essentially relational. I have long argued that we need to promote not care, but caring relationships (Herring 2013). Caring is a two-way process. Good care is, in its nature, relational. The two parties engage in a deep interchange in which the separation between carer and cared for breaks down. There is giving and receiving; a mingling of bodies; a breaking down of boundaries. The rich literature on ethics of care emphasises the values of attentiveness, responsiveness, respect, and mutual responsibility as being at the heart of care (Herring 2013). Yet these values and this deeply relational understanding of care is lost when care is seen as a commodity that can be bought and sold, where it is a service which can be selected from the cheapest provider. Personal budgets claim to put P in charge, but potentially lose long-standing caring relationships between patients and professionals.

There is a danger too that that if care simply becomes something available on the market – a commodity with a price – it leads to a downplaying of our individual responsibilities towards those with whom we are in relationships with. It also overlooks the collective responsibility we all have to those in our community who have particular needs. Our relationships generate particular personal obligations, and they cannot necessarily be met by simply purchasing a replacement (O'Rourke 2014). In particular, the marketisation creates the danger that care will be seen as the responsibility of those who chose to take on the job of carers, rather than recognise it is an inevitable and important part of everyone's lives. As Rummery (2011: 139) puts it:

> Caring relationships are often complex, involving reciprocal ties and obligations which are linked to both the emotional and physical aspects of providing and receiving care. Formalising and policing such arrangements run the risk of pulling apart the interlinked components of an ethic of care.

Not only does marketisation fail to appreciate the emotional aspect of care, but it also overlooks the importance of time in caring: the unpredictability of a caring relationship; being available as needed; for keeping apart; drawing together. All of this does not fit into a time sheet or a thirty-minute time slot. The continuity and reliability of care is lost (Lewis and West 2014). This is not to say that "budget driven care" is worthless, but we should realise and acknowledge its severe limitations. It is true that these concerns arise similarly when care services are supplied by a local authority. However, the explicit transfer of care needs into a finite sum of money in the context of personal budgets exacerbates this tendency to "box in" care.

The importance of relational care is all the more important given the huge issues surrounding loneliness among some older people and other socially excluded groups. It has been claimed that 1 in 10 older people feel chronically lonely all or most of the time (Campaign to End Loneliness 2017). There are complex reasons for this, but one may be the depersonalisation and marketisation of care. When caring is presented as simply a job that can be valued in market terms and can be replaced by whatever service is the cheapest, the relational value is severely challenged.

Another aspect of this is that as we meet the care needs of people by putting them in charge of their own budgets, we endanger the communal response to needs. Day care centres, local authority communal activities, and other social activities are lost because we have individuals seeking separate services, rather than a local authority seeking what services to provide for service users in their area. As George Monbiot (2014) has put it, 'the market was meant to emancipate us, offering autonomy and freedom. Instead it has delivered atomization and loneliness'.

Notes

1 Section 32 sets out when an adult without capacity can receive direct payments, at the request of an authorised person.
2 Care and Support (Personal Budget Exclusion of Costs) Regulations 2014

References

Audit Commission, 2008. *Guidance on Personal Budgets*. London: Audit Commission.
Barnes, M., 2011. Abandoning care? A critical perspective on personalisation from an ethic of care. *Ethics and Social Welfare*, 5(2): 153–167.
Baxter, K. and Glendinning, C., 2013. The role of emotions in the process of making choices about welfare services: The experiences of disabled people in England. *Social Policy and Society*, 12(3): 439–450.
Campaign to End Loneliness, 2017. *Threat to health*. London: Campaign to End Loneliness.
Carers UK, 2011. *Choice or chore?* London: Carers UK.
Carr, H. and Hunter, C., 2012. Are judicial approaches to adult social care at a dead-end? Care as a problem space. *Social and Legal Studies*, 21: 73–98.
Clements, L., 2008. Individual budgets and irrational exuberance. *Community Care Law*, 11: 413–428.

Collins, J., 2014. The contours of vulnerability. *In* J. Herring and J. Wallbank (eds.) *Vulnerabilities, Care and Family Law*. Abingdon: Routledge, 22–53.

Department of Health, 2007. *Putting people first*. London: Department of Health.

Department of Health, 2010. *A vision for adults social care*. London: Department of Health.

Department of Health, 2011. *Factsheet 4: Personalising care and support planning*. London: Department of Health.

Department of Health, 2014. *Care Act 2014: Statutory guidance*. London: Department of Health.

Department of Health, 2017. *Adult social care market shaping*. London: Department of Health.

Ferguson, I., 2007. Increasing user choice or privatizing risk? The antinomies of personalization. *British Journal of Social Work*, 37: 387–412.

Glasby, J. and Beresford, P., 2006. Who knows best? Evidence-based practice and the service user contribution. *Critical Social Policy*, 26(1): 268–284.

Glendinning, C., 2007. Increasing choice and control for older and disabled people. *British Journal of Social Work*, 37: 1335–1349.

Glendinning, C., 2008. Increasing choice and control for older and disabled people: A critical review of new developments in England. *Social Policy & Administration*, 42, 451–476.

Glendinning, C. et al., 2008. *Evaluation of the individual budgets pilot programme*. London: IBSEN.

Glendinning, C. et al., 2009. *The individual budgets pilot projects: Impact and outcomes for carers*. York: University of York.

Glendinning, C., Mitchell, W. and Brooks, J., 2014. Ambiguity in practice? Carers' roles in personalised social care in England. *Health and Social Care*, 23(1): 23–32.

Hamilton, S. et al., 2016. The role of family carers in the use of personal budgets by people with mental health problems. *Health and Social Care in the Community*, 25(1): 158–166.

Hatton, C. and Waters, J., 2013. *The second POET survey of personal budget holders and carers 2013*. London: Think Local Act Personal.

Her Majesty's Government, 2012. *Caring for our future*. London: The Stationery Office.

Herring, J., 2013. *Caring and the law*. Oxford: Hart.

Herring, J., 2014a. *Relational autonomy and family law*. Amsterdam: Springer.

Herring, J., 2014b. The disability critique of care. *Elder Law Review*, 8: 1–17.

Ismail, M. et al., 2017. Do personal budgets increase the risk of abuse? Evidence from English national data. *Journal of Social Policy*, 46(2): 291–311.

Kelly, D., 2013. Editorial: Reflecting on the implications of the Care Act 2014 for care providers. *Journal of Care Services Management*, 7: 74–79.

Keywood, K., 2003. Gatekeepers, proxies, advocates? The evolving role of carers under mental health and mental incapacity law reforms. *Journal of Social Welfare and Family Law*, 25: 355–375.

Leece, J., 2004. Money talks, but what does it say? Direct payments and the commodification of care. *Practice: Social Work in Action*, 15: 211–234.

Lewis, J. and West, A., 2014. Re-shaping social care services for older people in England: policy development and the problem of achieving 'good care' *Journal of Social Policy*, 43 (1): 1–18.

Manthorpe, J. and Samsi, K., 2013. 'Inherently risky?': Personal budgets for people with dementia and the risks of financial abuse: Findings from an interview-based study with adult safeguarding. *British Journal of Social Work*, 43(5): 899–903.

Mickel, A., 2008. What's the outlook for adult social care? *Community Care*, 23 Oct., 28–30.

Mitchell, W. and Glendinning, C., 2016. Allocating personal budgets/grants to carers. *Journal of Social Work*, 44(8): 2272–2289.

Monbiot, G., 2014. Sick of this market-driven world? You should be, *The Guardian*, 5 August. Availaible from www.theguardian.com/commentisfree/2014/aug/05/neoliberalism-mental-health-rich-poverty-economy (last accessed 22 October 2017)

Morris, J., 2003. *Barriers to independent living*. Leeds: University of Leeds.

Needham, C., 2011. *Personalising public services: Understanding the personalisation narrative*. Bristol: The Policy Press.

O'Rourke, G., 2014. Older people, personalisation and self: An alternative to the consumerist paradigm in social care. *Journal of Social Policy*, 43(1): 1–18.

Owens, J., Mladenov, T. and Cribb, A., 2016. What justice, what autonomy? The ethical constraints upon personalisation, Ethics and Social Welfare. *Ethics and Social Welfare*, 11(1): 3–18.

Pollock, A., 2005. *NHS PLC: The privatization of our health care*. London: Verso.

Poole, T., 2007. *Direct payments and older people*. London: King's Fund.

Rummery, K., 2011. A comparative analysis of personalisation: Balancing an ethic of care with user empowerment. *Ethics and Social Welfare*, 5(2): 138–151.

Schwehr, B., 2016. Your questions answered on direct payments under the Care Act. Available from: www.communitycare.co.uk/2016/10/11/questions-answered-direct-payments-care-act/ [Accessed 21 June 2017]

Slasberg, C., Beresford, P. and Schofield, P., 2013. The increasing evidence of how self-directed support is failing to deliver personal budgets and personalisation. *Research, Policy and Planning*, 30(2): 91–105.

Social Care Institute for Excellence, 2011. *Budgets and beyond*. London: SCIE.

Social Care Institute for Excellence, 2012. *Personalisation: A rough guide*. London: SCIE.

Spandler, H., 2004. Friend or foe? Towards a critical assessment of direct payments. *Critical Social Policy*, 24: 187–203.

Stewart, A., 2005. Choosing care: Dilemmas of a social market. *Journal of Social Welfare and Family Law*, 27: 299–317.

Ungerson, C., 2004. Whose empowerment and independence? *Ageing and Society*, 29: 189–205.

Williams, F., 2001. In and beyond new labour: Towards a new political ethics of care. *Critical Social Policy*, 21: 467–489.

Wood, D., 1989. Care of disabled people. Available from: www.psi.org.uk/publications/archivepdfs/Disability%20and%20social/WOOD.pdf [Accessed 21 June 2017]

Woolham, J. et al., 2016. The impact of personal budgets on unpaid carers of older people. *Journal of Social Work*, 33: 1–22.

6 "More than my job is worth" – defensive medicine and the marketisation of healthcare

Anant Jani and Andrew Papanikitas

An introduction to defensive medicine

In British slang, a 'jobsworth' is a term of abuse levelled at someone who refuses to help you because it will jeopardise his or her employment in some way. 'Jobsworth' is an abbreviation of, "It's more than my job is worth." Often it is applied to those who will not exceed their remit, even to a small degree, in providing assistance or who slavishly follow protocol when it is clearly inappropriate. Healthcare professionals are not immune to 'jobsworth' behaviour. Defensive medicine arguably represents a kind of 'jobsworth' behavior, dependent on a notion of protecting the livelihood, reputation or even the perceived conscience of a healthcare professional in preference to attending to the needs of any particular patient.

> Defensive medicine refers to medical care performed primarily to reduce the risk of litigation.
>
> (Bishop and Pesko 2015)

Defensive medicine is a phenomenon that has increasing prevalence across healthcare systems globally and can generally be divided into two categories:

> Positive defensive medicine, or assurance behavior, occurs when unnecessary services (i.e. diagnostic tests, procedures, referrals) are provided to patients to reduce the chance of patients taking legal action against a physician. Negative defensive medicine, or avoidance behavior, occurs when physicians refuse to provide high risk procedures and/or provide care to high risk patients.
>
> (Bishop and Pesko 2015; Studdert et al. 2005; Antoci et al. 2016)

Defensive medicine presents a clear and present danger to good healthcare and as such ought to be resisted. It is unquestionably a fact of current medical life. Several studies have pointed to the increased role defensive medicine is playing in how physicians and surgeons deliver care:

- A study of 800 doctors in Pennsylvania highlighted that 92% were ordering diagnostics procedures for assurance and 42% avoided high risk patients and/or procedures.

  (Rothberg et al. 2014)

- Between 2001 and 2005, 50% of A&E doctors in California acknowledged that their practice was influenced by concerns about malpractice lawsuits.

  (Sekhar and Vyas 2013)

- A study of over 100 gastroenterologists in Japan identified concerns about lawsuits as a driver for decisions they made about care.

  (Sekhar and Vyas 2013)

- A 2014 study revealed that 28% of over 4000 test procedures were at least partially defensive in nature.

  (Rothberg et al. 2014)

- 2,000 U.S. orthopaedic surgeons were surveyed and 96% agreed they practiced defensive medicine; furthermore, the study also highlighted that 24% of tests were ordered for defensive reasons.

  (Sethi et al. 2012).

While it is difficult to definitively measure whether any particular test or procedure, or lack thereof, was done for defensive reasons, it cannot be denied that the practice of defensive medicine has had a significant and adverse impact on global healthcare systems. Defensive medicine increases the financial costs of healthcare delivery, decreases the quality and safety of healthcare and reduces access to healthcare. This is because unnecessary tests and interventions increase costs in and of themselves, and false positive results may stimulate further anxiety and further tests. Many tests are also invasive in nature, and complications as a result of unnecessary tests compound the problem with costs incurred not only in treating those complications but, paradoxically, any litigation resulting from the defensive behaviour. Defensive medicine also reduces access to healthcare if waiting lists increase because of the larger number of tests and procedures being done. Access is reduced if physicians practice avoidance behaviour because the sickest and most difficult to treat patients are likely to have the worst outcomes (Rothberg et al. 2014; Hermer and Brody 2010).

In this chapter, we will consider how defensive medicine both influences and is influenced by a healthcare market. We will do this by considering why defensive medicine is bad for healthcare. We will consider the influence of marketisation on defensive medicine and of defensive medicine on markets. Finally, we consider some of the proposed solutions. In this chapter, we talk of physicians and doctors interchangeably, largely referring to all medically qualified clinicians but noting that the papers we cite use the term to mean medically qualified hospital doctors rather than surgeons or general/family practitioners. Of course, defensive medicine need not be a purely medical phenomenon, and we invite the reader to consider how other clinicians, managers, administrators and lawyers employed by healthcare institutions might engage with it.

1. The role of stakeholders and the effect of the market on defensive medicine

> For us, the deeper issue is [that] modern medicine has become driven a lot by technology, a lot by money – and we need to free decisions to be driven by patients' needs. – Vikas Saini.
>
> (Packer-Tursman 2015)

When considering the evolution and spread of defensive medicine it would be easiest to place the blame directly on doctors trying to avoid risk and/or opportunistic lawyers, but this would be a gross oversimplification. The key stakeholders in the healthcare system (patients, physicians, payers and other private sector stakeholders such as the medical technology sector and the legal profession) have had, and continue to have, an important role in the propagation of defensive medicine. Below we highlight some of the factors that have played a role in these different stakeholders supporting the evolution and spread of defensive medicine. Reviewing these factors, the reader will notice that they originate in mechanisms designed to make medicine safer, of a higher quality and more efficient.

1.1 Patients

We firstly consider patients as end-users of healthcare. Whilst even those who do not pay directly may feel that they pay through taxation or insurance, we find it helpful to distinguish entitlement to healthcare from direct purchase of it. Moreover, healthcare has perennially claimed to be an ethical activity aimed at patient benefit, even altruism (Glannon and Ross 2002).

The ostensible shift away from paternalistic medicine has meant a greater drive towards transparency of clinical decision-making and attention to patient education. While this has obvious benefits, it has also had the unintended consequence that patients, sometimes only partially instead of fully-informed, make demands, sometimes unrealistic, of their clinicians about treatments and interventions. Indeed, a study in 2005 highlighted that pacifying demanding patients was a key reason for medical specialists to go through the process of ordering costly tests and interventions.

> People come in wanting antibiotics, wanting studies, wanting to see the specialists . . . – Kisha Davis, medical director of Casey Health Institute.
>
> (Antoci et al. 2016)

Further, patients are able to communicate more freely with each other via online fora and social media, which makes it easier to compare relative care delivery. While this is definitely an important development, it has also contributed to patients making comparisons with each other of the care they are receiving. This has raised patient expectations and has also decreased patient tolerance for errors – both of which drive patients to more readily sue doctors if they feel they did not receive the standard of care they were expecting (Adwok and Kearns 2013).

1.2 Doctors

There are several ways in which physicians and surgeons have directly contributed to the rise of defensive medicine.

The most well-recognised and documented mechanism that has driven physicians to contribute to the propagation of defensive medicine is their fear of lawsuits from patients and their relatives. A 2013 study demonstrated that physicians who had the greatest concern about malpractice lawsuits were much more likely to engage in defensive medicine practices (Carrier et al. 2013). This concern is, unfortunately, also validated by data. A study published in the *British Medical Journal* in 2015 showed that for physicians across six separate specialties, higher spending on tests and procedures was associated with reduced malpractice claims (Jena et al. 2015).

A very important contributor to the persistence of defensive medicine is the presence of perverse financial incentives, particularly in fee-for-service systems, for physicians to order more tests and/or interventions because it leads them to earn more money (Hermer and Brody 2010; Lefton 2008). Further pressure for physicians comes from patients who demand tests and interventions, which may not be clinically indicated. If physicians do not meet their patients' expectations for standards of care, there is a risk that their reputation will suffer (Antoci et al. 2016). Reputation loss may also mean that patients who can seek healthcare elsewhere will do so and relationships with other payers may also be adversely affected – in effect reputational loss may mean loss of 'business'.

Physicians working within defined clinical pathways or standards of care established within their institution, usually established with the intention of standardizing care and/or reducing the risk of malpractice, will often not have the ability to make judgements on a case by case basis about tests and/or interventions for individual patients. This may lead to patients getting tests and interventions they do not actually need (Hermer and Brody 2010). Doctors and other clinicians may be reluctant to deviate from clinical guidelines, even where clinical acumen suggests that these are inappropriate, because clinical guidelines approximate a responsible body of medical opinion. In other words they approximate standard practice. The 'responsible body of medical opinion' is a legal standard by which a doctor may be judged in a court of law – and deviation from such orthodoxy needs to be justified – something which doctors, especially those in training or unfamiliar with a test or treatment, may lack the confidence to do.

1.3 Payers

Two key contributions payers have made in the propagation of defensive medicine is the use of fee-for-service payment mechanisms and, for insurance-based payers, having widely inclusive insurance policies. Both of these mechanisms give physicians a perverse financial incentive to over-test and over-treat their patients. (Sekhar and Vyas 2013) As Roland has outlined, however, any payment structure can offer perverse financial incentives (Roland 2012). There perhaps ought to be a broad similarity between how patients are treated in an insurance-based healthcare system and a state provided one – in both cases there are finite resources and inappropriate tests and treatments ought to be discouraged. Even here there is a dilemma for individual clinicians who need to strike a balance between the harms of routine testing and the harm of missing a diagnosis, such as cancer, where early diagnosis might make a difference to patients.

1.4 The medical technology sector

Technological advances in medicine have driven huge improvements in the delivery of safer and higher quality care in the twentieth and twenty-first centuries. Rapid improvements in technology have also helped to reduce the per-test and per-intervention costs in many cases. Both of these sets of factors have also made it easier for clinicians to order tests and interventions for patients, which has been a great contributor to defensive medicine (Adwok and Kearns 2013). Whilst individual tests are cheaper and more accessible, their aggregate consumption has the potential to be a greater expense. Above we have mentioned as well that tests are not harm free – a key harm being the possibility of a false positive result, or a failure of the test to reassure (McCartney 2017).

1.5 Lawyers

The group that is singled out as the biggest contributor to the rise of defensive medicine is lawyers. Amongst lawyers as a group, those who are blamed are the lawyers that act on behalf of patients in suing healthcare providers. In thinking about the role of the legal system in medicine we cannot downplay the important role it has played in making medicine safer by holding medical professionals accountable for avoidable medical errors and reckless behavior. Like the other factors highlighted in this section, however, the checks and balances provided by the legal system to ensure safer care have mutated into a system which often has opportunism at its core leading to unnecessary lawsuits and unregulated damage awards, which has had the effect of making doctors practice medicine in a more defensive way to protect themselves (Studdert et al. 2005). These behaviours are not unjustified – for example, most U.S. surgeons face malpractice claims in their career, and there is a 70% chance they will need to make an indemnity payment (Antoci et al. 2016).

   In this section, we attempted to highlight how the evolution and spread of defensive medicine is much more complicated than a phenomenon driven by the behavior of risk-averse doctors and/or opportunistic lawyers. All of the key stakeholders in the healthcare system have had an important role to play in the establishment of defensive medicine, often times through factors that were also essential in making medicine safer, of a higher quality and more efficient.

2. The effect of defensive medicine on the healthcare market

Some aspects of defensive medicine may not be driven by purely economic considerations – notable examples of concepts that drive defensive medicine being reputation and accountability. However, any system of exchange of goods for services is arguably a form of market, and in the following section we note the irony that a type of dysfunctional behaviour that is enhanced by market systems has a deleterious effect on those very same systems.

The most basic definition of marketisation in healthcare is the exposure of healthcare to market forces, which are the forces affecting the availability, demand and price of healthcare. From this definition, it is clear that defensive medicine has had a profound effect on the availability, demand and cost of healthcare.

One of the clearest means by which defensive medicine affects demand is through a greater use of tests and interventions linked with assurance behaviour. Depending on the test or intervention in question, the increase in demand can sometimes lead to innovations that will lead to improved safety, quality and efficiency of the test or intervention. Often times, however, the increased demand will further affect the availability and price of healthcare. If the increase in demand due to assurance behaviour is not met with a corresponding increase in supply, a natural consequence will be decreased availability of healthcare services, which often manifests itself as delays to care and longer waiting lists. This phenomenon of decreased availability is particularly true for tests and interventions that need specialist input.

With respect to avoidance behaviour, the links between defensive medicine and availability are fairly clear – physicians refuse to deliver care to patients they deem too risky. This has a number of ramifications. As we mentioned above it is often the sickest and neediest patients who are also the riskiest and availability of care to those people may suffer. In the 1960s, Tudor-Hart famously articulated the inverse care law (Tudor-Hart 1971), that those most in need of healthcare may be the least likely to receive it. Defensive medicine could well be one of those factors that deter clinicians from addressing the needs of the poor and disenfranchised. Not only may their health be poorer at the outset but social barriers may interfere with effective following of medical advice and consequently outcomes may be poorer. Moreover, doctors' decisions may be consciously affected by such reflections (Bernheim et al. 2008). Conversely, maintaining a clientele that is healthy, perhaps by playing upon their anxieties or offering the latest 'fountain of youth' has the potential to cause harm through the offer of unnecessary intervention. Selecting the easiest cases erroneously inflates a reputation for success, and may even obscure the fact that a clinician is not as excellent as they claim to be. A frequent accusation levelled at the for-profit healthcare sector in the UK is that it 'cherry picks' the most straightforward cases (Allen and Jones 2011). This potentially has an effect on current and future care: It unjustly increases the burden of harder cases on those who conscientiously see all comers. Moreover, those cases that would be deemed straightforward enough to be seen by clinicians in training instead form the basis of a predictable workload aimed at generating a financial profit in the short term. Avoidance behaviour therefore is a potent potential source of injustice, but also has the potential to distort markets in healthcare. This last point is because risky and therefore unpopular work becomes ever more expensive, or its availability dwindles.

A barrier to defensive medicine is provided by the so called 'medical defence organisations' in the UK and medical malpractice insurers elsewhere. Clinicians pay a membership fee or premium so that these organisations will pay the legal costs of defending their reputations or compensate patients for harms resulting from negligent practice (where possible). Whilst there are differences between indemnity and insurance from the purchaser's perspective, all doctors in the UK, at the very least are required to have either one or the other as a condition of employment. As aspects of practice become more litigious and are deemed riskier, the cost of medical defence increases. This cost is not always borne by institutions and another worrying trend on the availability/supply side is the trend of physicians taking early retirement or stopping practices because of unaffordable defence organisation fees or malpractice insurance. (Adwok and Kearns 2013) This has recently been seen in out-of-hours general practice care in the UK. Rising costs of indemnity and insurance have made out-of-hours work economically unsustainable for GPs (NHS England 2016).

Defensive medicine's impact on both the demand on, and consequent availability of, healthcare has an obvious impact on cost. For tests that do not require specialist input, increased demand has led to a decrease in the cost per test which can be acknowledged as a positive effect on the overall cost of healthcare. However, the increase in the actual number of tests done for any given patient have, on the whole, increased the cost of healthcare. For tests and interventions that require specialist input, the increases in cost have been quite stark particularly because there has not been an increase in the supply to meet the increased demand. Layered on top of both factors, the increase in malpractice insurance premiums for physicians has meant that the cost of physician input has also increased. The overall effect has been that the cost of healthcare has dramatically increased because of defensive medicine practices (Anderson 1999).

> Health care is not and cannot function as a rational market. Much of the time, people just cannot purchase health care in the coolly deliberative, rational way they shop for a house or a car. When someone's doctor tells her that the lump she felt is malignant, she cannot defer treatment the way she might postpone buying a new spring wardrobe or a trip to the islands.
>
> (Hoffman 2015)

It is important to note that the marketisation of healthcare does not necessarily mean that it would drive healthcare towards operating as a true and rational market. For healthcare to function as a true and rational market would require that patients first had full knowledge 'symmetry', i.e. a thorough understanding of the technical nuances of the healthcare options available to them; and second they would need a wide variety of options to choose from (Antoci et al. 2016). Healthcare systems across the world are trying to move in this direction but no system is there yet and debate still rages as to whether this is a good direction in the first instance. For example, influential ethical models of the consultation advocate symmetry of purpose rather than full knowledge symmetry (Emmanuel and Emmanuel 1992). Cursory attempts at the knowledge symmetry (where information is made available without meaningful support to interpret it) are viewed as forms of abandonment of care or abdication of responsibility (Heath 2003).

Paradoxically, many of the factors that could drive healthcare towards operating as a true market are the same factors, highlighted above, that are contributing to the spread of defensive medicine and a corresponding marketisation of healthcare.

- Well-informed patients are a key factor in ensuring healthcare operates as a true market but, as previously highlighted, when patients are only partially informed, they make demands on their physicians about tests and interventions which may be unnecessary.
- Physicians work within prescribed guidelines, protocols and pathways with the intention of standardising care and reducing variation. However, this sometimes has the unintended effect of patients getting unnecessary tests and interventions because the physician feels that he/she lacks the autonomy to make a case-by-case decision about their patients
- The evolution of medical technology has helped medicine make huge strides in improving diagnostic accuracy as well as safety, quality and efficiency. Yet, at the same time, the wide availability of a variety of medical technologies has made it easier for physicians to order these procedures, and it has also raised expectation on the part of patients to have access to these tests and interventions.
- The presence of the legal system and the recourse patients have to the legal system in case of medical error is an essential check to hold physicians accountable for avoidable medical error and negligent behaviour, with the ultimate hope that this would contribute to better standards of care. However, the use and abuse of the legal system with respect to healthcare has contributed greatly to healthcare moving further away from functioning as a true and rational market. Furthermore, there is no evidence that fear of lawsuits has actually reduced the rate of medical error (Antoci et al. 2016; Packer-Tursman 2015) and it may actually lead to harm because it prevents stakeholders from having an open dialogue about errors and learning from their mistakes (Studdert et al. 2006).

The factors that could lead healthcare to operate as a true and rational market (and as a result to increase its quality, safety and value) are the same factors that are driving defensive medicine. This key understanding of the situation has important implications for how the healthcare community might work together to utilise these factors to facilitate, rather than hinder, healthcare system improvement.

3. Conclusion: is defensive medicine unavoidable?

Defensive medicine has evolved and been propagated by factors that are dependent on the evolution of the rest of the healthcare system. As highlighted above, several factors that are essential for the improvement of healthcare systems constitute a double-edged sword that has also contributed to the evolution and spread of defensive medicine. The future of defensive medicine will depend on how these factors are used by different stakeholders in the system. If we hope to control the spread of defensive medicine, stakeholders will need to work together to ensure that these factors are used to contribute to healthcare system improvement rather than the spread of defensive medicine.

Many initiatives are under way to stem the spread of defensive medicine and below we highlight five general mechanisms healthcare systems are using to improve healthcare and reduce the impact of defensive medicine. These approaches appear simple, but sadly they are not – and we highlight some difficulties with them. We nonetheless suggest they merit investigation.

1   *Reducing the stigma around medical errors:* Fostering mechanisms that reduce the stigma and disincentives around reporting errors would help doctors shift away from assurance and avoidance behaviour in their practice. It could help to create a culture where open communication about errors could be used to help physicians improve their practice and improve the safety of healthcare delivery. A critical component of this would be to include patients in the conversations about errors. Adwok and Kearns 2013)

2   *Re-establishing trust between the doctor and patient:* "If you want to fix defensive medicine, develop trusted therapeutic relationships using effective communication skills and be available to patients, period" (Packer-Tursman 2015). Fear of lawsuits dramatically hinders open discussion between physicians and patients, and this has the effect of eroding trust. Open discussion between doctors and patients about errors will help to re-establish trust and decrease the tendency for patients to sue when medical errors do occur (Adwok and Kearns 2013; Sirovich et al. 2011). The drive to create more open discussion between physicians and patients is the basis for the Choosing Wisely campaign in the U.S. (ABIM Foundation 2017) and the RCGP Standing Group on Over-diagnosis in the UK (RCGP Standing Group on Overdiagnosis, 2016), which highlight tests and interventions that provide little value to patients so that patients and physicians can together make rational and effective care choices and move away from defensive medicine.

3   *Modifying financial incentives and payment models:* It is important to remember that assurance behaviour is not driven solely by fear of lawsuits (Sethi et al. 2012; Hermer and Brody 2010); in fee-for-service models physicians also have a perverse incentive to do more tests and interventions even if their patients do not need them. It is well recognised that tort reform will need to occur alongside modifications to financial incentive structures, and one means of doing this may be to shift away from fee-for-service models to capitated and patient/population-outcomes based models (Adwok and Kearns 2013; Sirovich et al. 2011). Having said this, we are aware that any way of paying for services can be subject to gaming without appropriate regulation and ethical behaviour on the part of the service provider.

4   *Tort reform:* There is evidence that malpractice liability reforms are able to reduce pressures on physicians to use assurance and avoidance behaviour (Kessler and McClellan 1996). Furthermore, reducing stigma around medical errors and fostering more open discussion with patients could allow more

disputes to be resolved through mediation and arbitration rather than through litigation (Adwok and Kearns 2013).

5   *Modifying liability:* Modifications to medical liability have also been shown to reduce defensive medicine practices. For example, shifting liability from individual physicians to the healthcare institution in which he/she works and/or limiting the non-economic damages that can be awarded to patients can help to limit assurance and avoidance behaviour on the part of the physician (Antoci et al. 2016; Adwok and Kearns 2013). In the UK, NHS work carried out in NHS hospitals is indemnified by the State. Nonetheless, hospital doctors are obliged to make their own medico-legal indemnity arrangements. This is because institutions are considered to be more attractive targets for lawsuits on account of having more resources with which to settle claims. Institutions also have an interest in maintaining their resources and reputation, and this may create incentives to place blame back on clinicians. Worse still, defensive medicine may be adopted in institutional policy as well as in individual practice.

Through this analysis we have seen that defensive medicine contributes to marketisation and marketisation contributes to defensive medicine. However, defensive medicine actually prevents healthcare from functioning as a true and rational market. Paradoxically, we see that the factors that contribute to defensive medicine are also essential for the improvement of healthcare systems and are also important in helping healthcare to function as a true and rational market. It may be that for a market in healthcare to work, better understanding is needed of the economic irrationality alluded to in the quotation from Hoffman above (Hoffman 2015). If the defensive medicine phenomenon teaches us anything it is that there is a parallel irrationality on the part of the healthcare provider! It may be that defensive medicine and its marketisation effects represent a transition state that is unavoidable and necessary for healthcare to evolve into a rational market; the full conversion may only occur when the factors spreading defensive medicine are used to improve healthcare systems. One may also conclude, however, that it is too simple to lay both the blame and the solution with society's tools for safe and high-quality healthcare. Any tool requires responsible and adept use. As we have suggested above, the solutions may not always be simple – potentially involving both change to regulation and education, with a robust approach to both science and values. It is clear that defensive medicine is a present and clear danger to healthcare quality and patient safety, and as such must be addressed. An understanding of healthcare and of markets is of clear relevance to this task. The practice of good, safe and effective medicine should be intrinsic to healthcare and all of its stakeholders and, we suggest, not 'more than anyone's job is worth'.

References

ABIM Foundation, www.choosingwisely.org/ (accessed on 13/03/2017).
Adwok, J., and Kearns, E.H. (2013) Defensive medicine: Effect on costs, quality and access to healthcare. *Journal of Biology, Agriculture and Healthcare* 3: 29–35.

Allen, P. and Jones, L. (2011) Diversity of healthcare providers, Chapter 2, pp. 1–29, in *Understanding New Labour's Market Reforms of the English NHS*, The King's Fund, London, www.kingsfund.org.uk/sites/files/kf/chapter-2-diversity-health-care-providers-new-labours-market-reforms-sept11.pdf (accessed 01/08/2017).

Anderson, R.E. (1999) Billions for defense: The pervasive nature of defensive medicine. *Archives of Internal Medicine* 159: 2399–2402.

Antoci, A., Fiori Maccioni, A., and Russu, P. (2016) The ecology of defensive medicine and malpractice litigation. *PLoS One* 11: e0150523.

Bernheim, S.M., Ross, J.S., Krumholz, H.M., and Bradley, E.H. (2008) Influence of patients' socioeconomic status on clinical management decisions: A qualitative study. *Annals of Family Medicine* 6: 53–59.

Bishop, T.F., and Pesko, M. (2015) Does defensive medicine protect doctors against malpractice claims? *BMJ* 351: h5786.

Carrier, E.R., Reschovsky, J.D., Katz, D.A., and Mello, M.M. (2013) High physician concern about malpractice risk predicts more aggressive diagnostic testing in office-based practice. *Health Affairs* 32: 1383–1391.

Emmanuel, E., and Emmanuel, L. (1992) Four models of the physician-patient relationship. *Journal of the American Medical Association* 267: 2221–2226.

Glannon, W., and Ross, L.F. (2002) Are doctors altruistic? *Journal of Medical Ethics* 28: 68–69.

Heath, I. (2003) A wolf in sheep's clothing: A critical look at the ethics of drug taking. *British Medical Journal* 327: 856.

Hermer, L.D., and Brody, H. (2010) Defensive medicine, cost containment, and reform. *Journal of General Internal Medicine* 25: 470–473.

Hoffman, D.R. (2015) The effect of patient demands and defensive medicine on health care costs. *Philly.com*, 26 February. Web.

Jena, A.B., Schoemaker, L., Bhattacharya, J., and Seabury, S.A. (2015) Physician spending and subsequent risk of malpractice claims: Observational study. *British Medical Journal* 351: h5516.

Kessler, D., and McClellan, M. (1996) Do doctors practice defensive medicine. *The Quarterly Journal of Economics* 111: 353–390.

Lefton, R. (2008) Addressing roadblocks to hospital-physician alignment. *Healthcare Financial Management* 62: 30–31.

McCartney, M. (2017) Benefits, harms and evidence: Reflections from UK healthcare, Chapter 2, pp. 11–16, in *Handbook of Primary Care Ethics*, Eds. Papanikitas, A. and Spicer, J., London: CRC Press.

NHS England (2016) GP Indemnity Review, www.england.nhs.uk/wp-content/uploads/2016/07/gp-indemnity-rev-summary.pdf (accessed 01/08/2017).

Packer-Tursman, J. (2016) The defensive medicine balancing act. Web blog post. *Medical Economics*. Modern Medicine, 9 January. Web.

RCGP Standing Group on Overdiagnosis (2016) Report to RCGP Council, www.rcgp.org.uk/policy/rcgp-policy-areas/overdiagnosis.aspx (accessed 01/08/2017).

Roland, M. (2012) Incentives must be closely aligned to professional values. *British Medical Journal* 345: e5982.

Rothberg, M.B., Class, J., Bishop, T.F., Friderici, J., Kleppel, R., and Lindenauer, P.K. (2014) The cost of defensive medicine on three hospital medicine services. *JAMA Internal Medicine* 174: 1867–1868.

Sekhar, M.S., and Vyas, N. (2013) Defensive medicine: A bane to healthcare. *Annals of Medical and Health Sciences Research* 3: 296–296.

Sethi, M.K., Obremskey, W.T., Vatividad, H., Mir, H.R., and Jahangir, A.A. (2012) Incidence and costs of defensive medicine among orthopedic surgeons in the United States: A national survey study. *American Journal of Orthopedics* 41: 69–73.

Sirovich, B.E., Woloshin, S., and Schwartz, L.M. (2011) Too little? Too much? Primary care physicians' views on US health care. *Archives of Internal Medicine* 171: 1582–1585.

Studdert, D.M., Mello, M.M., Gawande, A.A., Gandhi, T.K., Kachalia, A., Yoon, C., Puopolo, A.L., and Brennan, T.A. (2006) Claims, errors, and compensation payments in medical malpractice litigation. *New England Journal of Medicine* 354: 2024–2033.

Studdert, D.M., Mello, M.M., Sage, W.M., DesRoches, C.M., Peugh, J., Zapert, K., and Brennan, T.A. (2005) Defensive medicine among high-risk specialist physicians in a volatile malpractice environment. *JAMA* 293: 2609–2617.

Tudor Hart, J. (1971) The inverse care law. *The Lancet* 297: 405–412.

7 Covenant, compassion and marketisation in healthcare

The mastery of Mammon and the service of grace

Joshua Hordern

> No one can serve two masters, for either he will hate the one and love the other, or he will be devoted to the one and despise the other. You cannot serve God and Mammon.
>
> (Matthew 6:24, ESV)

1. Serving and measuring[1]

'No one can serve two masters . . . You cannot serve God and Mammon.' Jesus' famous words, cited to different purposes by Miran Epstein and Adrian Walsh in this volume, provide a starting point for this chapter's constructive argument and critical conversation with the chapters in this middle part. Epstein deploys Jesus' words to deny the possibility of any constructive reconciliation between capitalism and healthcare, contrasting Jesus' saying with the infamous words of Christian conquistadores and with what he claims is the inherently corrupting, master-slave ethic of the Deuteronomic covenant. By contrast, Walsh cites Jesus to explain Judeo-Christian cultural suspicions about money's place in healthcare before delineating the potentially, *though not necessarily*, corrosive effects of marketisation.

Jesus' teaching suggests that determining what *mastery* and *service* mean is central to any ethically and culturally sophisticated interpretation of marketisation's multiple influences amidst the suffering which healthcare is instituted to address. Accordingly, the core insight to be taken from Feiler's and Herring's criticisms of concrete examples of marketisation within health and social care may be summarised as follows: that which we serve will be determined in part by the representation of ourselves and our neighbours to which we subscribe. Certain representations of care and of work are perpetuated by concrete forms of marketisation within health and social care, such as those Herring and Feiler explore. Values embedded within certain kinds of codification and budgetary policy master the consciousness of patients and healthcare workers. These values' effects on human relationships seem to Herring and Feiler inimical to the ethos which ought to mark the practice of health and social care.

In my view, the representations of self- and neighbour-care and of work which follow from such mastery are necessarily of political significance since the healthcare institutions affected are those upon which political self-consciousness in part depends. My questions follow:

- What image of health and social care work is in fact represented by the specific cases of marketisation that Feiler and Herring have critiqued?
- What kind of political story should be told about citizens by the processes of marketisation which affect their health and social care? How *should* people and their caring relationships be represented?
- How should Christian pastoral and political theology answer these last two questions to enable judgments to be made between benign and malign forms of marketisation?

Critique of the representations of health and social care is an essentially pastoral and political activity. Everyday experiences of care, requiring pastoral sensitivity, are influenced by system-wide developments. Such pastoral sensitivity must also be political, informed by insight into political conditions, narratives and beliefs which shape people's lives.

The Archbishop of Canterbury, Justin Welby, analyses late liberal economic and political life in this spirit. For Welby, what is measured has come to be what matters. 'Mammon draws our gaze away from things that are more worthy of our attention but have not been given the badge of a comparable monetary value' (Welby 2016, p. 40). In short, 'what we measure controls us' (ibid. p. 35). Those worthy of our attention and service are neglected. That which we create as a quantifiable standard of success comes to master us.

This pastoral concern finds a desultory echo in the effects of a target culture on care among staff in the British NHS. As McCann et al observed in relation to one institution:

> [the] targets regime was forcing [staff] to try to please two masters, and in the process incentivizing them to move in two very different directions. A middle manager in the ambulance trust explained this in a very simple phrase: "You can't do both – something will give".
>
> (McCann et al. 2015, p. 784)

The consequences for institutional morale are unsurprising:

> [the] kinds of goal displacement inscribed in the attitude of "what's measured is what matters" . . . remains pervasive within the NHS. Other failings, distortions, and forms of "gaming" . . . create perverse outcomes and typically result in a decline in morale for public service professionals.
>
> (ibid. p. 777)

I will argue that *covenantal* modes of thought and practice, native to Jewish and Christian thought in their representations of human life, are peculiarly sensitive to that which tends not to be represented in the marketisation processes to which Feiler and Herring pay attention. Accordingly, following (1) these introductory remarks explaining my approach I will (2) now engage critically with the ways that care and work are represented in Herring's and Feiler's chapters. Then I will (3) build on this to develop a constructive, pastoral-political proposal focussing on the themes of covenant and compassion in order to address the issues of service, mastery, history, personalisation and responsible choice which surround processes of marketisation before (4) coming to a conclusion.

2. The representation of care and work

To articulate how covenantal thinking dethrones Mammon in practice, it will be helpful first to reflect on the challenges which have been analysed by Feiler and Herring. These will be categorised under two themes which define both chapters' underlying rationale.

2.1 Care

The commodification of care inherent in the codification of Diagnosis Related Groups and the use of personal budgets represents, most fundamentally, a risk to the *representation* of care. That kind of risk is fundamental because the core of a culture is formed by its loves, by the ways it comes to value that which it shares. But that which is valued, loved and shared is defined by what people perceive – what is represented to the self and to the community as true about the world. Hence the risk of a false representation of care. Will what is measured so master care as to distort what ought to define the relations between persons?

DRGs, on Feiler's account, have been a chief instrument in a 'transvaluation' now embedded in ways of perceiving healthcare which simultaneously entrench and cleverly conceal from criticism the representations of the patient-as-consumer and healthcare-as-product to be delivered. A more extreme underlying transvaluation is that the patient becomes represented by the cash value of their care need – an end obscenely demoted into a mere economic means.

In manifold subtle ways, patients are made to follow or serve the money, illustrating in interpersonal relations the mastery by Mammon which Jesus warns against. However, rather than giving in to an apparently uncontrollable evolutionary process, understanding the historical processes in which marketisation occurs makes dethroning Mammon possible.

The insight of pastoral and political theology is that none of Hayek's three kinds of order which account for the development of any particular state of affairs – *taxis*, *kosmos* and *catallaxy* – have any regard to what Christian theology has learned to call the moral order of creation to which all 'orders of love' are called to correspond in order to enable truthful perceptions of neighbours and to restrain the distortion of care. By this account, it is a person's or institution's order of love which shapes and directs the compassion which characterises that person or institution (Hordern 2013a; cf. Hordern 2013b; Hordern 2017).

This sharpens the question of what might sustain regard, make perception truthful, restrain distortion and order compassion aright. For Feiler, the ultimate consideration is the plenitudinous, generous gift of God in Christ which enables a steady polemic against and resistance to any conflation of healthcare with the logic of a market committed to the maximisation of utility and the extraction of profit. This is clearly in some tension with Petratos (2018), who has a positive and subtle approach to utility considerations in healthcare.

Personal budgets, for Herring, encourage the perception of care as a commodity to be bought and sold. The devolution of choice to the individual, intended to liberate people in their personal autonomy, becomes that by which people are enslaved, especially in their doubts, fears and worries. To put it in more sinister terms, the patients' 'value' precisely as sources of income is 'liberated' *to* the play of market forces.

To elaborate Herring's analysis, observe that the state, in this devolutionary process, may 'retail' certain interpretations of liberation by disseminating stories about its citizenry. One such is the tale Herring reports of the woman we might call 'Dancing Sally' who, disentangled from the leaden-footed, stumbling state, is free to jig at all hours, supported by her lively personal assistant, funded by her personal budget. Care is represented here as supporting a joyful exodus from the loneliness and inactivity which an inflexible, state-dominated, depersonalised system can impose. The policy which inspires this representation aims to energise vibrant local markets which can individually service the diverse needs of clients who choose to deploy their personal budget. The patient-as-consumer becomes the master of her care, not the servant of the constricting choices of others.

Herring, however, draws on empirical studies to paint a less than flattering picture of how this policy has created a diminished image of care with desultory effects on people's lives. Potentially negative emotional experiences have indeed been transferred to 'service-users' – a concrete example of the 'relocation' about which Feiler is concerned. For one study from the evidence Herring cites, the

> implication [of the research], that people who feel negative whilst making welfare-related decisions tend towards avoiding rather than embracing these decisions, is important, especially within the context of policies that assume choice is beneficial *per se* and that opportunities for choice should be maximised.
>
> (Baxter and Glendinning 2013, p. 448)

Herring and I share a fundamental concern to support caring relationships (indeed who could disagree with this?). But my question is whether some framework for the 'personalisation' of social care, within a suitably diversified market, well-populated with prospective employees, underpinned by the guarantee of state action for those unwilling to participate in the market directly, can support the development of a caring, compassionate polity. This is to some degree in tune with the principal positive claim of Petratos (2018), namely that the decentralisation of healthcare enables services to be better fitted to people's preferences.

The evidence suggests that, for many, the benefits of taking control over personal budgets is principally a matter of timing. As one contented citizen in a study to which Herring refers said:

> I've got my head round everything else. It's all dealt, it's all slotted into its own place, and now direct payments is a doddle. It just does not seem like a problem now. But then it did, and I wouldn't touch [it] with a bargepole because it just seemed so much work and so much time and effort.
>
> (ibid p. 446)

So finding the right time to take control by entering the market is important. But time is also a key factor in relationships between carer and 'service-user'. For another study Herring cites, we learn that, rather than being inherently damaging to caring relationships,

> [carers'] psychological well-being was significantly associated with having a regular arrangement for someone to take care of the service user to enable the carer to have a break.
>
> (Glendinning et al. 2009, p. 79)[2]

More ambiguously perhaps, the study also reports that

> carers reported that a service user's ability to pay a carer could contribute to positive outcomes for the IB [individual budget] user by reducing feelings of dependency and indebtedness.
>
> (ibid. p. 94)

Just what is negative about dependency and indebtedness is not itself analysed. Perhaps it was the sense of being a burden on society and relatives, in which case the 'positive' quality of the outcome would be contested by those who believe that care is learnt through acknowledging interdependency.

Nonetheless, it is clear that direct payment for care, personalised in this way with responsibility given to those who wish to have it and with the availability of a suitably trained care workforce, can make for *some kind of* emotional contentment and provide much-needed relief. It is not obvious that state or local authority monopoly control of social care provision is in any way better fitted to deliver 'positive' outcomes.

The Baxter/Glendinning study summarises the overall position well by concluding with the moderate, practical observation that the evidence does not support 'an argument against devolving responsibilities, but for empowering people by offering appropriate support in all aspects of making choices' (Baxter and Glendinning 2013, p. 448).

The core problem which emerges from Herring's analysis concerns how the 'relational autonomy' he commends should interrelate with the degree of control exercised by the state or local authority, bearing in mind policy trends towards personalisation, choice and responsibility (personal, familial and charitable). Addressing this problem is vital when discerning whether and how caring may be well represented in marketised health and social care environments.

2.2 Work

The *work* involved in health and social care is also represented in certain ways in DRGs and personal budgets. Feiler cites Maio's view that the industrialised, standardised, hyper-efficient processes have increasingly robbed healthcare professionals of a patient, conscientious, compassionate, joyful and authoritative sense of vocation. The human freedom to do good work before God upon which a humane healthcare system depends is distracted and mastered by economic technocracy. For Herring, the logic which orders the personal budgets system cements a debasement of caring work by ignoring the nature of caring relationships. What seems to be necessary, therefore, are ideas and structures which fortify resistance to this debasing of professionalism (Roland 2012). A reassertion of vocation remains prone to failure if it is not interwoven within a socio-political consciousness, fully informed about the historic nature of developments in healthcare marketisation.

However, personal budgets clearly affirm the valuable personal work of taking care of oneself and shaping the caring relationships one enjoys. It is perhaps too easy to point to those who lack the ability to do so and for whom personal budgets are not appropriate either at all or at this time or in an unsupported fashion. Herring himself observes that no one is compelled to pursue a personal budget approach. While compulsion comes in many forms, the fact that only 5% said that they felt pressured to do so seems a vindication of the approach, considering the potential vulnerability of those who use the service.

By contrast, the positive opportunity for some citizen-patients to share responsibility seems a significant benefit. While the pastoral care of those who feel unfitted – either always or at a particular point in time – to take such responsibility could no doubt be improved, it seems hard to deny that the work of self-care, in a supportive environment, is not empowering for some, perhaps for many or even most. The empirical evidence does not rebut this claim.

What Feiler and Herring agree is that care work is inadequately represented in the forms of marketisation they examine. Herring does not recommend dismantling the entire personal budget system, noting that it is a mixed picture in terms of outcomes. Feiler, one imagines, would welcome the liberation of healthcare from DRGs. However, her practical recommendations turn more in a diakonic direction, thus following Petratos' approach rather than Herring's (Petratos 2018, p. 29; Feiler 2018, p. 29; Herring 2018, p. 93). These critiques do not tell against any and every kind of marketisation, but they do issue a strong exhortation that the possible effects of marketisation in some circumstances should be mitigated, held in check or reversed.

What seems necessary are modes of resistance to demoralisation – to the consciousness becoming mastered by processes associated with marketisation. The central goal should therefore be to uphold better representations of care and work to resist debasement and strengthen what is good. In the third part, therefore, I will now turn to think about how this goal can be pursued.

3. Covenant and compassion

Mammon's mastery of healthcare relationships is to be resisted. But what kind of political story should be told by and about citizens to dethrone Mammon in the processes of marketisation which affect their health and care? How *should* people, their caring relationships and their work of care, be 'represented' in specific policy approaches? What will sustain regard, guide perception into truth, restrain distortion and order compassion aright?

The kind of representation in view here differs in an important respect from those analysed in respect of Feiler and Herring. Rather than being an unselfconscious *misrepresentation* of care on account of marketisation processes, the *covenantal* mode of representation to be explored below enables judgments to be made *between* benign and malign forms of marketisation. When representation of health and social care relationships are normatively presented within a 'covenant', a certain kind of story about who people are and how they ought to relate is told.

3.1 Almsgiving and ordered loves

The long traditions of Jewish and Christian reflection on covenant and wealth offer wisdom here. John Chrysostom, the fourth-century church father, taught that almsgiving is a powerful weapon to break the power of wealth which can master us, binding us like a chain. The way to conquer wealth, Chrysostom argues, is to distribute it: when we are isolated it binds us – 'but when we bring it forth among others, it will master us no more, holden as it will be in chains, on all sides, by all men' (Chrysostom 1839, p. 177). For Chrysostom, people are to master money by being bound together rather than being mastered and bound by it, in isolation from each other. This is not an argument against money itself as he says: 'God made nothing evil, but all things very good; so that riches too are good . . . if they do not master their owners' (ibid. p. 177). This is what 'despising' and 'hating' (Matthew 6:24) means in practice – an orientation and practice which is so conscious of the quasi-divine draw of Mammon that it requires Mammon's submission to God, 'whose service is perfect freedom' (Church of England).

For this Christian tradition, almsgiving bears witness and responds to the prior generous initiative of God, giving freely that humanity might not be enslaved to Mammon. There is a relational wisdom in the *manner* of God's acts of salvation which climax in the gift of Christ incarnate, crucified, risen and ascended. God's initiative invites participation in a new and covenantal mode of relating between God and humanity and among human persons – ways of being bound together through ties of grace, binding the power of other things to enslave us.

This covenantal wisdom lies uniquely in the mode of gracious initiative which calls forth a faithful and free response to break with Master Mammon. As Justin Welby puts it:

> Dethroning Mammon requires the dramatic leap of faith of being defined by what we do not measure – cannot measure – because it is the infinitely valuable, utterly cosmos-transforming love of God in Jesus Christ.
>
> (Welby 2016, p. 57)

The new covenant in Christ binds its parties together in a manner which both guarantees their future relationship and requires daily, responsible choices on the part of the recipients of grace. The nature of the covenant tells a certain kind of story about those who trust the promise of God which initiates the covenantal relation. They become conscious of the dangers which surround their journey through life – that wealth can master and bind their personal and institutional consciousness and practice.

On a systematic level, Rusthoven comments that its

> central position in redemptive history and its relational character make the covenant theme well suited as the basis for a normative understanding of relationships within creation, including those that form in the course of medical practice and research.
>
> (Rusthoven 2014, p. 186)

That which provides the normative structure of God's redemptive work in Israel and in Christ is in no way dissonant from the created order. In other words, God vindicates his creation through his redemptive work.

In vindicating it, God provides the basis for the benign relational life of caring Herring commends, and the distortions of perspective in DRGs which Feiler rejects. It is neither the *cosmos* nor *taxis* nor *catallaxy* of Hayek, but rather the created order of God, vindicated in Christ, which should discipline human relations within a certain order of love (*ordo amoris*). This order takes a specific form in covenantal modes of loving relations between God and human persons and among those persons, modes which bind money's power by graciously inspiring obligations for self and others, guiding vision and informing compassion.

While almsgiving by a church, structured by this specific mode of covenantal thinking, has a rationale which is distinct from the way that funds for health and social care are codified and dispersed in a plural society through taxation, there are nonetheless observations which may be made by interrelating these modes of handling money through the theme of covenant.

First, far from being a judgment on those outside the new covenant and in a striking example of critical self-awareness, it is the *church* which Chrysostom warns about the temptations that arise in the context of money. In short, covenants should operate to dispel complacency about money and foster self-criticism of ways in which its presence in relationships provides opportunity for self-deception and temptation.

Second, almsgiving in the church's story provides a core practice for preventing the distortions which inordinate attention to wealth and money can introduce. The practice is intended to represent the generosity of God by reflecting it, thereby fulfilling the purposes of the new covenant life into which the church was born. To be a faithful participant in a covenant is both to show trust in the God of the covenant and, only through the economy of grace that this God enacts, to become a trustworthy partaker of it by working to serve one's neighbours, especially with one's wealth. In this way, care and work are enfolded within the terms of the covenant that is enacted between God and the church and which forms a point of resistance to the service of Mammon against which Jesus warns.

With typical wisdom, Rabbi Sacks makes the congruent point that covenant has a power of a quite different order than money. Whereas, if 'I have a thousand pounds and share it with nine others . . . I am left with a tenth of what I had', when I share certain kinds of goods such as friendship, kindness or love, I end up with more not less. The secret to this strange economy is to cultivate 'environments in which we are bound to one another not by transactions of power or wealth but by *hessed*, covenant love . . . God lives in *the between* that joins self to self through an act of covenant kindness' (Sacks 2005, p. 54; cf. Sacks 2000).

In similar ways, specific practices of health and social care will embody certain ways of either enabling covenant love or entrenching distortions of desire. Because of humanity's creation in the image of God within an orderly creation, mutuality, love and obligation are to mark such practices and the institutions the practices sustain. This is the basis for the possibility of the caring relationships Herring and Feiler – in their different ways – commend. Well-framed covenants give order to loving relationships within creation, thereby shaping the compassion that characterises persons and institutions.

3.2 Covenant and marketisation

This is not at all to suggest that it is inevitable that once 'covenant' is invoked, then money's mastery will be no more, bound by the covenant love and compassion in terms that Chrysostom and Sacks would commend. Not all summons to a covenantal mode of thinking and relating are equally illuminating.

For example, Rusthoven pays no sustained attention to marketisation's significance for a covenantal ethic in medicine. Commercial exploitation is discussed briefly only in relation to Islamic bioethics (Rusthoven 2014, p. 94). It is perhaps the lack of attention to the granularity of covenantal relations (e.g. between God and Israel) that led to this oversight, and it is an object lesson for any reference to covenant in health- and social care.

By contrast, William May, the forefather of twentieth-century covenantal thinking in healthcare, was explicit that the core rationale for thinking in covenantal terms is the threat to medical professionalism presented by marketisation. He identified the influence among U.S. doctors of increasingly commercialised representations of care in a minimalist, contractual way of conceiving relations between doctors and patients. While a legal contract has a proper place within healthcare to protect patients or doctors in some circumstances, it may introduce distortion when professional relations are reduced to the level of commercial contracts alone. (May 1975, pp. 33–35). In particular, a mere commercial-contractual model misses out on the 'element of the gratuitous' (ibid. p. 35) which covenants involve and the moral obligations which covenanting parties have towards each other.

In 1995, the drafters of the *Patient-Physician Covenant* gave further content to covenantal thinking by specifically targeting a 'growing legitimation of the physician's materialistic self-interest ... [and] for-profit forces [pressing] the physician into the role of commercial agent to enhance the profitability of health care organizations' (Crawshaw et al. 1995; cf. Misselbrook 2018, pp. 148–153).

For both May and the covenant drafters, covenantal language in some way reaches beyond normal human relations. Cassel, a co-author of the covenant, writes of a 'transcendent significance to the activities of healing', noting that while 'the physician's role in the lives of patients may not be godlike or divine, at its best it can and ultimately does have spiritual dimensions' (Cassel 1996, p. 605).

May is more theologically explicit than this somewhat anaemic reference to the 'spiritual', observing 'the secret root of every gift between human beings, of which the human order of giving and receiving could only be a sign' (May 1975, p. 35). With attention more granular than Rusthoven's, to the farming practices of Ancient Israel and their significance for sharing in the common wealth of the nation, May observes that the

> ethic of service to the needy flowed from Israel's original and continuing state of neediness and indebtedness before God. Thus action which at a human level appears gratuitous, in that it is not provoked by a specific gratuity from another human being, is at its deepest level but gift answering to gift.
>
> (ibid. p. 36, cf. Hordern 2013a)

Thus Israel, in their own internal practices, represents the gift they receive and so, ideally at least, model a life of gracious initiative.

This focus on obligation to others stemming from grace, articulated as a covenant which is closely attentive to economic realities, functions to sensitise May to the range of obligations at stake in a covenant specifically concerned with healthcare. He criticises the nineteenth-century American Medical Association's tendency to allocate 'duties' to physicians but 'obligations' to patients, not because it is improper to talk of patients' obligations but because the notion of doctors' duties as stated under-realised doctors' profound indebtedness to their society – with its universities and hospitals – and to their patients, who are willing to assist in their education, thereby providing the environment in which medical students could be trained and realise a useful social vocation (May 1975, pp. 31–32).

However, the *Patient-Physician Covenant* lacked this rooted granularity and omitted any attention to the obligations of patients and society or of the rationale for physicians' obligations to society, focussing solely on the 'covenant of trust with patients' as fulfilled by physicians. Cassel explains that central to the Covenant's rationale is 'the perceived threat . . . to the sacred responsibility of physician to patient. The Covenant was crafted as a call to renew medicine's commitment to the core mission of concern for the sick and thus to maintain the soul of the medical profession' (Cassel 1996, p. 604). While the seed of the thought of a well-rounded perspective on obligation is clearly there in the Covenant, it has not come to maturity.[3]

By contrast, May's attentiveness to the range of obligations is rooted in a perspicuously Christian covenantal consciousness of the nature of love: 'not that we loved God but that he loved us' (1 John 4:10; May 1975, p. 36). For May, this recognition of the prevenient love of God both in an individual and across a society has concrete implications. Specifically, it generates an awareness of that which comes before our agency in the world, of that which we receive from others. In particular, this leads to a focus on the inherited nature of the societal conditions which enables physicians to flourish and which creates a sense of the reciprocal obligations that physicians and patients have with each other.

Such an awareness circumscribes the consciousness which doctors might have in entering a market for their services. The lack of balance between obligations which emerge in a condescending paternalism that pretends to a self-sufficient medical profession, free in the marketplace, is addressed by a covenantal sense of all of life as a gift from God, which is mediated through civilised ways of ordering life devised by humans and passed on to each succeeding generation. This does not rule out participation in selling one's services but makes such participation answerable to prior creaturely obligations.

On these two points, the granularity of the attention to economic realities and a focus on the obligations of all parties – especially those inherited by doctors – it is precisely the focus on specifically Jewish and Christian sources of covenantal thinking that makes May's account compelling. It is then to a fine-grained focus on specific kinds of covenant that we now turn.

3.3 Comparing covenants

Covenants, if well-framed, represent truthful ways of describing the relations between persons. Their pastoral strength and capacity to generate compassion lies in this kind of relational sensitivity. They can also tell a certain kind of political and economic story about a polity of citizens, whether that be ancient Israel or a modern nation-state. Parties to the covenant are made aware of the range and source of the obligations they have, the blessings they enjoy and the risks to those blessings if obligations are not fulfilled. By discerning obligations, blessings and risks within an historical narrative, attentive to hard-won institutional achievements that make possible a certain kind of civic life in which healthcare has a central role, the apparent inevitability of marketisation's mastery of human desires is challenged.

For Christian theology, it is precisely the historic nature of God's engagements with the creation in love, through Israel, Christ and the church, which sensitises people to such a covenantal consciousness. Covenantal thinking impels a critical engagement with the kind of story which has been told about the responsibilities and forms of gratuitous love and compassion which mark a relationship, a profession and a polity of citizens.

A well-framed covenant thus represents a certain kind of story based on how ecologies of mastery and service have come to evolve in any given culture, laying the basis for reappraisal, critique and resistance to 'inevitability' if a story has developed in a way which no longer enhances sharing in certain goods and wise debate about their nature and use. As stated earlier, "that which we serve will be determined in part by the representation of ourselves and our neighbours to which we subscribe". These self-understandings may change over time. Covenants have a peculiar capacity to challenge and to reorder such change.

A parallel which demonstrates the power of covenantal thinking to represent work, care and obligations and to shape self-understanding is the UK Armed Forces Covenant, referred to in the UK Armed Forces Act (2011).[4] A key source of inspiration for the Armed Forces Covenant described how

> mutual obligation forms the Military Covenant between the Nation, the Army and each individual soldier; an unbreakable common bond of identity, loyalty and responsibility which has sustained the Army throughout its history.
>
> (UK Ministry of Defence 2000)

The Covenant pays particular attention to these mutual obligations which government representing society and service personnel owe to each other. The armed forces' obligations are focussed on tasks which they commit to fulfil, often at significant risk, in bearing arms and undertaking other politically authorised activities. Societal and governmental obligations are focussed on the welfare of service personnel and their families in light of the risks to which they are exposed and sacrifices which they make on behalf of their nation and other nations.

For both parties, there is an element of gratuity which goes beyond anything a contract can require: the obligations owed to the armed services are supported by, but never entirely exhausted by, specific legal provisions. Creativity is needed to discern how best to fulfil the covenant at the social and moral level, especially in terms of according respect and honour to armed forces personnel and families. The obligations owed by members of the armed services are distinctively gratuitous in that they in principle commit to hold nothing back, even their lives.

Healthcare services also involve sacrifice and risk, even risk to one's own life, albeit to a lesser extent. Though the bullet-wound and needle-stick injury differ in the scale of risk they pose, there is nonetheless a shared exposure to threats undertaken on behalf of others. Where health is nationalised, both forms of service represent a nation inasmuch as the work which they do and the loving care with which they do it tells a certain kind of story about the identity of a polity and what it may require of its people. Both have, for many years at least, warranted respect and honour to those who provide them.

Not for nothing are the armed services central to UK national celebrations and commemorations. Not for nothing was the National Health Service at the heart of the 2012 London Olympic opening ceremony. And not for nothing do failures to keep covenant by healthcare staff (e.g. surgical misconduct) and armed forces personnel (e.g. extra-judicial killings) strike at the core of the national psyche, causing a breach in existing covenantal relations, whether tacit or explicit. Both sets of professionals embody forms of service which are central to the contested story the United Kingdom tells about itself and which becomes explicit when the occasion requires that the nation becomes self-conscious. These professions' very institutional lives represent a kind of self-image to which the nation is summoned to debate and defend.

Just how sacrifice and risk figure in the service represented in these institutions of national life of particular importance to the devising of any prospective healthcare covenant. The obligations inherent in the Armed Forces Covenant focus squarely on the welfare of armed services personnel and their families in light of the risks they face. Because of the nature of the work which the armed forces do, this is entirely appropriate. The extreme sacrifice which energises the mutuality that is the background assumption of the Covenant is the basis for this concern for welfare.

Any prospective healthcare covenant would not be so straightforwardly focussed on the welfare of health and care workers and their families, even bearing in mind the risky possibilities of such work. Nonetheless, there are threats to human wellbeing which the profession of medicine commits a health or care worker to encounter. In such a covenant, when professionals and patients keep their mutual obligations, they keep them not just with each other but also with society as a whole, since the pains and costs of ill health are born not just by individuals but also, in some sense, by the whole community.

So it seems imperative that an emphasis on workers' welfare should be included both in covenantal thinking and in any written articulation of covenantal relations. Welfare in this case would pay attention especially to the form of the working conditions, the provision for dependents and the commitments of patients and managers to staff which are promised. Among armed forces personnel, *esprit de corps* and camaraderie are cemented by the extreme kinds of threats to their lives as well as those of others that they encounter together, commonly yielding remark-able regimental loyalties. Since, in healthcare, the normal threat is to *others'* lives, a key covenantal focus should be on the risk to workers' wellbeing, which encoun-ters with suffering and death on a nation's behalf engender.

In summary, the terms of a covenant and, crucially, the manner in which a covenant is implemented, tells a certain kind of story about a polity – what it values, what it loves, what sacrifices it will make and why it will be committed to maintaining those sacrifices amidst hardship. Just as the UK Armed Forces Covenant is intended to fit the specific nature of armed service in the context of a nation's historical circumstances, so also a Healthcare (or Health and Care) Covenant would fit the specific nature of healthcare service in the context of a nation's historical circumstances, reacting to certain problems and fending off certain dangers. The specific nature of a certain profession's work of care is the key determinant for the shape of any covenant. What is decisive is the kind of political story which a covenant tells, in its formulation, in its practical outworking and in the breach – when commitment to covenant fails.

Returning explicitly to our theme of marketisation, a covenant should stress that to be mastered by money threatens that desire for service which strengthens the self-understanding of a profession or nation. To serve Mammon as master puts pressure on the possibility of covenantal relations of care and work shaped by gratuity as opposed to solely contractual obligation. Government is a key broker in seeking to fend off the temptations which can attend the presence of money in covenantal relationships.

3.4 Five requirements for a healthcare covenant

What requirements should shape a Healthcare Covenant, written and owned by all parties, which attends wisely to the challenges and opportunities of marketisation? What covenantal provisions or emphases would sustain regard, guide perception into truth, restrain distortion and order compassion aright?

> **First, a healthcare covenant should deploy historical sensitivity in binding all parties together in order to bind the tendency to distortion of desire which accompanies money's presence.**

Distorted desires and modes of practice should be addressed by the articulation and institutional embodiment of certain deep commitments which both tell the truth about the development of a story and write a new and better chapter. On Feiler's view, the acceptance of DRGs has created a certain kind of ahistorical consciousness on the part of those who administer them, concealing the origins of the codification, making invisible the care of those who are codified and abandoning those same people to the drivers which the codification brings about. And yet, as Feiler comments, 'historically grown healthcare systems are *always already* the result of (potentially religiously grounded) truth commitments – anthropological, political, eschatological' (internal reference Feiler). The healing which healthcare requires is in part one which achieves the hope of reconciliation between those persons who have become hidden from each other, submerged beneath an apparently inexorable, never-ebbing tide of monetisation.

> **Second, the historic indebtedness of each physician, who is dependent on both patients and the existing healthcare infrastructure for training and for ongoing opportunities to perform meaningful work, should be basic to any covenant.**

This emphasis follows on but fills out some detail of Feiler's important but as yet somewhat abstract claims. Nigel Biggar makes a similar point in his perception of the debt of gratitude that each generation owes to that which precedes it, grounding a sense of obligation especially to one's nation (Biggar 2014). This is an important argument against conceiving healthcare staff as wandering healers-for-hire, a problem especially pertinent to doctors in underfunded state-run organisations such as the NHS. This dimension of marketisation is perhaps most damaging in the context of a socialised system such as the British NHS, in which significant taxpayer funding is deployed to subsidise doctors' training when their future employment by the state is not guaranteed.

Third, covenantal thinking implies responsibility-taking by all parties, including the patient, for their and others' welfare, including the welfare of healthcare workers.

May emphasises the image of the patient as 'active participant both in the prevention and the healing of the disease. He must bring to the partnership a will to life and a will to health' (May 1975, p. 36). For some, the personal budgets policy provided just the opportunity for that active participation and collaboration with health and care workers.

However, Rusthoven comments that the 'increased interest in covenantal models coincides with efforts to address the overemphasis on patient autonomy that has largely replaced traditional paternalism' (Rusthoven 2014, p. 136). Enraptured with an emphasis on purely self-sacrificial *agape* love as the basis of covenantal care as distinct from the reciprocal *hessed* Sacks commends, he claims that 'reciprocation should not be a necessary and expected outcome. The scriptural mandate to help others and to show mercy must remain in the foreground' (ibid. p. 256).

While it is true that despite 'human failure to maintain obedient obligations to that covenant, God has repeatedly shown his faithfulness to that covenant' (ibid. p. 260), 'the sacrifice and selflessness that mark a covenantal approach to health care' (ibid. p. 264) by no means entail the exclusion of the reciprocity that properly marks a healthcare covenant. Moreover, this means not only taking responsibility for one's own well-being but also, developing Herring's thought, that of those participating in a caring relationship with you. The parallel with the Armed Forces Covenant is particularly relevant here as a basis for societal obligations to partner with and ensure the welfare of healthcare workers as they encounter their neighbours' suffering and death. By contrast, 'defensive medicine', as discussed by Jani and Papanikitas (2018), represents a cultural aversion to, and abdication of, responsibility-taking in favour of self-protective practices, characterising not only clinicians but also whole institutions.

Fourth, while responsibility-taking is core to covenant, covenantal thinking must also be defined by grace and flexible enough to encourage discretion in individual circumstances.

Herring's rather critical approach to personal budgets surely has some traction here. The practical outworking of the scheme seems to have included at least something of the sense of being abandoned to one's own autonomy rather than the relational autonomy Herring commends. Some local authorities seem to have been glad to shift responsibility more or less wholesale – so to speak – from their institutions to citizens' shoulders, be they strong or weak. This is a general temptation which accompanies forms of marketisation that place the burden on the 'consumer' – *caveat aeger* ("let the sick person beware")!

Recalling John Chrysostom's concern to bind money's power in the church, what covenantal thinking highlights is the danger of leaving people isolated with responsibility for money – the hazard of a mere contract which is neither fitted to the person nor in any way gracious. Covenantal thinking encourages responsibility for the work of care to be distributed in a supportive way, specific to the person at hand.

Moreover, it is the ultimately non-contractual nature of the covenant which allows discretionary sensitivity to the capacities of the individual rather than an all-or-nothing requirement. While covenant involves gratuity, it also involves sensitivity to specific circumstances, making it so eminently suitable for a personalised healthcare which is underwritten and circumscribed by a covenanting community.

Honest conversation with patients about errors as recommended by Jani and Papanikitas (2018) would also be a feature of a gracious covenantal relationship. In the context of covenant, it is possible not only to take responsibility for errors in relation to individuals who suffer its effects but also to construe error in relation to community benefit. Processes for reporting error can be gracious towards health professionals' errors while candid with those affected. But these processes will work best if the relationship between healthcare professionals and society is not conceived solely in terms of contract, with its inbuilt logic of defensiveness and litigation, but primarily as a long-term learning covenant.

Fifth, a covenant must be explicit about the implications of failures to keep covenant.

In ancient Israel, one of the characteristics of the covenantal relationship between God and his people was the provision of curses which would come upon the people pursuant to their failures to be faithful and loyal (e.g. Deuteronomy 27–30). A curse amounting to a loss of honour represents the final words of the Hippocratic Oath.

A distinctive feature of any prospective healthcare covenant is most clearly seen when one considers that the penalties for failures in keeping obligations within a covenant are found in the consequences experienced by all concerned rather than in sanctions applied to any particular individual. In other words, failures in responsibility will often have significant social implications. Just as armed service is not private – or at least is never of private significance alone – so healthcare is not private – or at least is never of private significance alone. This is more explicit in a socialised health system in which a limited fund must cover the entire population's need. But even in a private insurance based system, it is clear that premiums payable will depend, to some degree, on the actions of all, and that bad outcomes to healthcare, while impacting individuals primarily, also have social ramifications.

In summary, a Healthcare Covenant should be psychologically astute about the historic context in which marketisation processes are operative; attentive to the historic indebtedness of health- and social care workers in order to challenge a pure free agent mentality; unembarrassed about the obligations of all parties, including patients' obligations for the welfare of themselves and their carers; full of grace and discretion when it comes to individual circumstances; and explicit about what follows from failures in covenant.

A covenant thus characterised will guard against the pendulum swinging between extremes of ahistorical consciousness/uncritical conservatism, marketised ultra-mobility/stultifying statism, autonomy/paternalism, pure self-sacrifice/merely contractual reciprocity and legalism/license. It does so by keeping the different kinds of responsibility bound together in a single, if contested, narrative, with a view to ensuring that money never masters but rather is mastered by a community of compassion and grace.

4. Conclusion: mastering Mammon, renewing compassion

Just as in the case of the contrast of Rusthoven and May, it would be an overstatement to suggest that an appeal to the notion of covenant is a *simple* solution to the systemic problems which Feiler and Herring identify in the concrete practices of marketisation that they consider. The outworking of the Armed Forces Covenant as a social or moral matter rather than a merely legal one bears witness to the challenges on the level of policy which covenants require.

What a well-framed, written, legally backed covenant can achieve is a stable sensitivity to the threats which would obscure or undermine the relationships of mutual obligation, embedded in specific practices of relational care, which the covenant seeks to preserve. A covenant explicitly makes visible and valorises these practices which constitute the institutions – such as hospitals, local authorities and providers of social care – which shape a people's civic life. These institutions are then the formal manner of representing in practice a covenant that restrains the love of money, makes visible those relationships which ought not to be obscured, denies the supremacy of choice in a market to the exclusion of care and articulates the architecture of obligation. Indeed, a covenant which is not enacted in practice is hardly worthy of the name. Through healthy, wise institutions, money may be mastered through the moral and social power of a covenant whose realisation binds money's power and brings to conscious awareness the persons with whom one is in promissory relations.

With respect to defensive medicine, Jani and Papanikitas (2018) judiciously lay out some of the policy approaches which could address the tendencies that undermine trust between doctors and patients. They are conscious that the pursuit of worthy goals can give grounds for entrenching defensiveness, and that any payment model, however carefully devised, is subject to abuse. What is required to direct goals and to cement trust is not only a wiser payment model and not only an emphasis on safety, quality and efficiency. More fundamentally, what is required is that healthcare relationships are conceived in a way which promise that the presence of Mammon will not overwhelm the encounter of persons which is at the heart of covenantal healthcare.

Such an approach in no way requires that covenants in respect to health and social care be solely formed on a national level or be restricted to relations between citizens and state institutions. Indeed, the focus of covenants on relationships which transcend the contractual would lend itself well to the more localised and personalised forms of care relations which personal budgets are meant to facilitate. That which can be captured in a commercial contract would very likely fall far short of what is required. Dancing Sally can contract for her assistant to put in the hours and take her to the dancehall. But she could hardly contract that her assistant dance the waltz with her on occasion, and still less, do so 'with feeling'.

In limiting the power of Mammon and its modes of measurement to influence ways of perceiving and caring for people, covenants reorder loves. That which draws attention away from the suffering of the persons for whom one is called to care is that which should be resisted through the terms of covenant. To reorder loves in service of those who suffer is to renew compassion. It is therefore a covenant of compassion which can resist the temptations which lurk within the marketisation process. Equally, it is a covenant of compassion which can guide that personalisation of care that properly serves individuals in their circumstances.

Accordingly, health- and social care professionals should seek to form and enter into covenants which bear witness to a certain kind of story about a compassionate common life. In the terms of a political and pastoral theology, the covenant between healthcare professionals and society should be in some sense a reflection of the covenant between God and his people – Israel and the church. This reflection will be imperfect because of the difference between the parties covenanting in the two cases. But there will also be a similarity inasmuch as the covenant is formed amidst suffering and over against the dangers of isolation and abandonment to lonely and arbitrary choice.

Such covenants are defences against the corrosive elements in healthcare marketisation processes which Walsh identifies (Walsh 2018). It is not that there is a total incompatibility between service and commercialisation, or indeed between serving and measuring. Rather, the question is which master is served and what money is made to follow. In the words of the Archbishop of Canterbury, it is a matter of making money serve grace. Some mix of moral persuasion and legal sanction is Walsh's recipe for moral rectitude. While this is welcome, it seems inadequate to shape healthcare work, especially when it is compared to the work of the armed services. A covenant based on gracious interrelations and the taking of responsibility seems best fitted to foster the sensitivity and resistance to corrosion for which Walsh hopes.

The relational life which a covenant envisages is properly called 'communion'. In the life of the church for whom Chrysostom preached, this was a holy communion, the life of the church set apart by God to resist Mammon's mastery. However, as I have explained elsewhere, the nature of communion in a plural political society is not holy but tense (Hordern 2014). Health- and social care institutions embody, at least in plural Western democracies, the meeting point of many different ways of communing in humanity's suffering condition. The specific terms of a covenant in a plural society, precisely because they require an internalised acceptance – a matter of the heart – cannot be those which necessarily require confession of faith in the God revealed in Jesus Christ. However, as I have argued here, a wise conception of a covenant which will aid health- and social care today, especially amidst the challenges and opportunities of marketisation, is best arrived at by drawing inspiration from Jewish and Christian sources of covenantal consciousness and compassionate practice.

Notes

1 Joshua Hordern's work is supported by the University of Oxford Wellcome Trust Institutional Strategic Support Fund (105605/Z/14/Z) and the Arts and Humanities Research Council (AH/N009770/1). The author gratefully acknowledges this funding and also that of the British Academy and the Sir Halley Stewart Trust. The views expressed are those of the author and not necessarily those of the Sir Halley Stewart Trust.
2 'Multivariate analyses of the structured interview data showed that IBs were associated with positive impacts on carers' quality of life, social care outcomes and psychological well-being. In relation to all these outcome measures, carers of IB users scored higher than carers of people using standard social care services; the difference between the two groups of carers was statistically significant in relation to carers' quality of life' (ibid. p. 89).
3 For example, it has been reaffirmed in its original form, by the American Psychiatric Association, in both 2007 and 2014. See www.psychiatry.org/File%20Library/About-APA/Organization-Documents-Policies/Policies/Position-2014-Patient-Physician-Covenant.pdf.
4 Different questions naturally arise regarding marketisation since there is nothing like the need for a state monopoly on healthcare provision when compared with the need for a near or total monopoly on the use of armed force, although there is a growing market for private armed contractors.

References

Baxter, K. and Glendinning, C. (2013). The Role of Emotions in the Process of Making Choices about Welfare Services: The Experiences of Disabled People in England. *Social Policy & Society* 12:3: 439–450.

Biggar, N. (2014). *Between Kin and Cosmopolis: An Ethic of the Nation*. Eugene, OR: Cascade.

Cassel, C. (1996). The Patient-Physician Covenant: An Affirmation of Asklepios. *Annals of Internal Medicine.* 124: 604–606.

Chrysostom, J. (1839). *The Homilies of John Chrysostom*. Oxford: Parker.

The Church of England (2017). *Book of Common Prayer*. Cambridge: Cambridge University Press.

Crawshaw, R., Rogers, D.E., Pellegrino, E.D., Bulger, R.J., Lundberg, G.D., Bristow, L.R. et al. (1995). Patient-Physician Covenant. *Journal of the American Medical Association* 273: 1553.

Feiler, T. (2018). Encoding Truths? Diagnosis-Related Groups and the Fragility of the Marketisation Discourse. In: Feiler, T., Hordern, J., and Papanikitas, A. (eds.) *Marketisation, Ethics and Healthcare: Policy, Practice and Moral Formation*. Abingdon: Routledge, pp. 67–83.

Glendinning, C., Arksey, H., Jones, K., Moran, N., Netten, A., and Rabiee, P. (2009). *The Individual Budgets Pilot Projects: Impact and Outcomes for Carers*. York: University of York/University of Kent.

Herring, J. (2018). Personal Budgets: Holding onto the Purse Strings for Fear of Something Worse. In: Feiler, T., Hordern, J., and Papanikitas, A. (eds.) *Marketisation, Ethics and Healthcare: Policy, Practice and Moral Formation*. Abingdon: Routledge, pp. 84–98.

Hordern, J. (2013a). *Political Affections: Civic Participation and Moral Theology*. Oxford: Oxford University Press.

Hordern, J. (2013b). What's Wrong with "Compassion"? Towards a Political, Philosophical and Theological Context. *Clinical Ethics* 8.4: 109–115.

Hordern, J. (2014). Loyalty, Conscience and Tense Communion: Jonathan Edwards Meets Martha Nussbaum. *Studies in Christian Ethics* 27.2: 167–184.

Hordern, J. (2017). Compassion in Primary and Community Healthcare. In: Papanikitas, A. and Spicer, J. (eds.) *Handbook of Primary Care Ethics*. London: CRC Press: 25–33.

Jani, A. and Papanikitas, A. (2018). "More Than My Job Is Worth": Defensive Medicine and the Marketisation of Healthcare. In: Feiler, T., Hordern, J., and Papanikitas, A. (eds.) *Marketisation, Ethics and Healthcare: Policy, Practice and Moral Formation*. Abingdon: Routledge, pp. 99–110.

May, W. (1975). Code, Covenant, Contract or Philanthropy. *Hastings Center Report* 5: 29–38.

McCann, L., Granter, E., Hassard, J., and Hyde, P. (2015). "You Can't Do Both – Something Will Give": Limitations of the Targets Culture in Managing UK Health Care Workforces. *Human Resource Management* 54:5: 773–791.

Misselbrook, D. (2018). The Virtuous Professional and the Marketplace. In: Feiler, T., Hordern, J., and Papanikitas, A. (eds.) *Marketisation, Ethics and Healthcare: Policy, Practice and Moral Formation*. Abingdon: Routledge, pp. 147–162.

Petratos, P. (2018). Why the Economic Calculation Debate Matters: The Case for Decentralisation in Healthcare. In: Feiler, T., Hordern, J., and Papanikitas, A. (eds.) *Marketisation, Ethics and Healthcare: Policy, Practice and Moral Formation*. Abingdon: Routledge, pp. 13–31.

Roland, M. (2012). Incentives Must Be Closely Aligned to Professional Values. *British Medical Journal* 345: e5982.

Rusthoven, J. (2014). *Covenantal Biomedical Ethics for Contemporary Medicine: An Alternative to Principles-Based Ethics*. Eugene, OR: Pickwick.

Sacks, J. (2000). *The Politics of Hope*. London: Vintage.

Sacks, J. (2005). *To Heal a Fractured World: The Ethics of Responsibility*. New York: Continuum.

UK Ministry of Defence (2000). *Soldiering: The Military Covenant*. London: Army Doctrine Publication, Volume 5.

Walsh, A. (2018). Commercialisation and the Corrosion of the Ideals of Medical Professionals. In: Feiler, T., Hordern, J., and Papanikitas, A. (eds.) *Marketisation, Ethics and Healthcare: Policy, Practice and Moral Formation*. Abingdon: Routledge, pp. 133–146.

Welby, J. (2016). *Dethroning Mammon: Making Money Serve Grace*. London: Bloomsbury.

Part III
The place of ethics

8 Commercialisation and the corrosion of the ideals of medical professionals

Adrian Walsh

Introduction

Over the past thirty years, medicine in the Western world has been subjected to market forces such that many medical practices – which were once governed by the State or by principles of gift – are now fully commercialised. Commercialisation here includes not only the buying and selling of goods which previously were not available on the market, but also the establishment of modes of analysis which regard all human interactions as fundamentally commercial in nature. Although there are undoubtedly advantages to such commercialisation, at least for some sectors of society, serious concerns have been raised about the effects on the proper ideals of medicine that the market leaves in its wake. In this chapter, I explore one such objection, the Corrosion Thesis, according to which the market corrodes our attitudes towards practices and entities that should be regarded as intrinsically valuable. I consider how various forms of commercialisation potentially corrode the ideals of medical professionals in ways that can only be harmful to practices of medicine and, ultimately, to the population at large. I focus on the Australian experience of commercialisation, and in particular the specific ways in which Australian medical practice has been commercialised, and how such commercialisation threatens valuable ideals associated with the provision of healthcare.

1. Commercialisation: definitions and policy responses

Let us begin by defining the term 'commercialisation' stipulatively. I shall use the term to cover three distinct, but related elements, these being:

(i)   *The commodification of goods and services* – that is the process whereby goods that were previously not commodities are transformed into entities that are bought and sold.
(ii) *The transformation of the method of distribution of goods and services* – that is, the adoption of market mechanisms to distribute and allocate goods.
(iii) *The application of economic modes of evaluation to healthcare practices and healthcare policies* – most notably, the use of cost-benefit analysis (and related methods) to determine choices between competing policies.

In general, the term 'commercialisation' will be used herein to denote the trans-formation of practices that were previously non-commercial into commercial practices; and in the medical sphere it denotes the commercialisation of medical goods and services.[1]

A central feature of commercialisation is a transformation of the incentive struc-tures associated with the production and distribution of social goods in which the *profit motive* becomes the organising principle of social life in commercialised areas. When a social good or practice is commercialised, those agents producing goods and services do so in order (in part at least) to make a profit. At the same time, the goods and services are distributed on the market with the producers aim-ing to maximise their profits. A consequence of this market allocation undertaken by profit maximising agents is that the question of who obtains the goods and services is determined by whomsoever can pay the prices that are consistent with the maximisation of profit for the producers. The profit motive is clearly at the heart of commercialisation.

In recent years in Australia there has been a great deal of pressure to com-mercialise the provision of medical goods and services (note that I will make use of Australian examples herein, but the points made are intended to generalise beyond the Australian context). Three significant examples spring immediately to mind. First, there has been the introduction of cost-benefit analysis to evaluate the relative merits of competing medical procedures and policies. Health policy, in general, is assessed in terms of the economic efficiency of the outcomes produced. Second, although there is a general commitment to the maintenance of a non-commercial public health system, governments in various states and at a federal level have implemented a two-tiered healthcare system in which a private system runs alongside the public health system. Those in the private healthcare system often gain preferential treatment and typically have better access to already scarce resources. The system in this sense has been *partially* commercialised. Third, there have been attempts to introduce a user-pays system for patients. This has been largely resisted for basic medical services – indeed the attempt by the then Abbott government to introduce co-payments for basic consultations was met with furious public outrage and was a factor in Abbott's downfall as Prime Minister. However, the gap between the coverage provided by Medicare and the fees charged by some medical practitioners is, in many cases, quite large.

These processes of commercialisation in medicine can be understood simply as cases of the general tendency towards commercialisation with market-based capitalist societies. In general, within Western societies there has been an increase in the range of goods available on the market and the extent to which social interac-tions are understood primarily in economic terms. Marx saw the expanding market as part of the need of capitalism to increase the so-called 'organic composition of capital', while the German social theorist Jurgen Habermas regards it as but one element in the 'colonisation of lifeworld'. At the same time as we note the general move towards commodification, it needs to be acknowledged that the historical processes have not been unidirectional; there have also been historical periods in which some goods and services have been de-commodified. The move, after the Second World War, in many Western democracies to establish public provision of healthcare services by the state represents one such significant moment of de-commodification.

There have typically been three main political responses to social processes of commercialisation. The first, which we might call *abolitionism*, involves (as the name suggests) abolishing market processes in response to what are regarded as the harms of the market and commercialisation. Marxism and various socialist movements would be prime examples of this position. The second – which might be referred to as either 'pro free-market' or 'libertarianism' – involves the wholesale endorsement of the market and all processes of commercialisation. Here market processes are regarded as socially beneficial or an expression of freedom, and hence their generalisation is regarded as an unquestionable good. The third political response, while permitting commercialisation, involves the regulation and constraint of trade by governments and relevant regulatory authorities to avoid harms that market processes are thought to pose. This we might label *regulativism*.

Notice that the third approach might also include preventing some exchanges in selective spheres of activity. So while the advocate of a regulatory approach might endorse commercialisation in many spheres of activity so long as it is properly regulated, such an advocate might also endorse what Michael Walzer called 'blocked exchanges', in particular *spheres* so that there are some goods that cannot be bought and sold (Walzer, 1983, p. 250).[2] This 'spheres' approach is evident in the medical sphere when we consider the ban in countries such as Australia and Britain on selling, for instance, human organs. The underlying thought here is not that markets in human organs need to be constrained by state regulation, but simply that they should not exist at all. One important message to take from this discussion is that it should not be thought that opposition to the commercialisation of medicine could only be understood in abolitionist terms.

2. The ideals of medical professionals

As professionals, there are a set of practices, standards and ideals to which medical personnel are expected to adhere. Community expectations involve the idea that medical professionals are committed to the healing of the sick and prevention of disease and of ill-health more generally. There is an expectation that the primary motivation should be towards the wellbeing of all members of the community, and conversely the producers should not overly focus on non-medical benefits such as wealth, prestige or power. A commitment to the wellbeing of the community is thought to bring with it a commitment to professional competency, compassion, respect and dedication.

One finds these expectations embedded in various medical codes and practice guidelines. For instance, the physicians' oath of the World Medical Association declaration of Geneva (1948) includes amongst other things a commitment to the idea that the health of the patient will be a physician's first consideration (Declaration of Geneva, 1948).

Australia's guide to Good Medical Practice – which was designed in 2010 to reflect the understanding of both the medical community and the public regarding the acceptable standards of professional conduct – provides an extensive list of duties (Epstein, 2018).[3] It talks of the professional beliefs and ideals the government and public expect medical practitioners to uphold. Amongst other things, the code says that they have the following obligations:

- *Provide good patient care*: including ensuring ongoing care, assessing patient and making decisions based upon this assessment, referring a patient to another practitioner
- *Maintain a high level of medical competence*: recognising limits
- Making decisions about health care is the *shared responsibility* of the doctor and patient
- Decisions about patients' access to medical care must be *free from bias and discrimination*.

(Medical Board of Australia, 2014)

The *Australian Medical Board Code of Conduct* notes that patients trust their doctors because they believe that "in addition to being competent, their doctor will not take advantage of them and will display qualities such as integrity, truthfulness, dependability and compassion" (Medical Board of Australia, 2014).

We can see a focus in all of these codes and guidelines on what the philosopher Alasdair MacIntyre calls the *internal goods* of a practice. Conversely, there is an expectation in many of them that medical professionals are not to be influenced by so-called *external* goods like money and power.

Note that some of these documents endorse not only the idea that these virtues are to be characteristic of medical professionals, but that they are *first virtues* of such professionals. John Rawls, in *A Theory of Justice*, famously argues that justice is the *first* virtue of social institutions and arrangements. By this, Rawls means that when there is a conflict between justice and other considerations such as economic efficiency, then justice should take precedence. Similarly, in some codes it is argued that the professional ideals of medicine always take priority when other duties and goals come into conflict with them. Take the "Declaration of Helsinki" (1948) as an example, with its demand that:

> the wellbeing of the human being should take precedence over the interest of science and society.

However, this is a much stronger claim than the initial claims that the medical profession has ethical obligations; and one can, of course, endorse the ideals noted above without 'buying into' the claim that they are the first virtues of medical institutions. It is also not clear that this is what the general public have in mind when it is argued that medical professionals have significant moral obligations, although of course that is not to suggest that closer inspection might not reveal some commitment to this gloss upon the idea of medical ideals.

The list put forward in the *Australian Guide to Good Medical Practice* provides, I suggest, a good overview of the kinds of ideals typically endorsed by both medical governing bodes and the public at large. Our question concerns the relationship between these ideals and commercialisation. How might these ideals be threatened by commercialisation? In the following sections, I shall outline some salient harms associated with commercialisation, before focussing on the Corrosion Thesis and how the harm of corrosion might impact upon the ideals stated above.

3. Objecting morally to the commercialisation of medicine

Why might one object to the commercialisation of medicine? Many people within contemporary society are extremely wary of the commercialisation of medicine. This dovetails neatly with the long tradition in political theory of treating the commercialisation of medical practices and medical resources with, if not outright hostility, great suspicion. We need only think of recent debates over the permissibility of commercial surrogacy or alternatively of the sale of human body parts to note the heated responses to proposals for more commercialisation that commercial medicine sometimes generates. This is part of a more general suspicion of commercialisation that has a long pedigree within Western culture. In part, this derives from the Judeo-Christian heritage that tells us that we cannot simultaneously serve God and Mammon, and in no lesser part from the writings of philosophers such as Plato and Aristotle for whom a commercial orientation was a sign of moral deficiency. The socialist tradition, of which Marx is perhaps the most well-known exemplar, regarded commerce as anathema and a site of corruption and exploitation.

It is worth, at this point, unpacking some of this hostility in order to identify reasons why one might object to commercialisation. Below I identify four such reasons before noting the objection most relevant to the ideals of medical professionals, namely the 'Commodification Objection'.

The first objection is the 'Distributive Objection' according to which commercialisation is morally pernicious because of the distributive consequences it has. Once goods are commercialised, then this means that they are typically allocated to those with sufficient funds to pay for them and, where goods are scarce, they are distributed only to those with the most money to pay for them. If the goods in question are basic needs – as many medical resources surely are – then it is a matter of injustice that one's access to these goods be dependent upon one's financial status.

A second commonly expressed objection concerns the exploitation (putatively) associated with the profit motive that is at the heart of commercialisation (Epstein, 2018).[4] On this line of reasoning, people who are motivated by profit must consciously or unconsciously exploit people from whom they seek to profit. Underpinning this is a zero-sum view of profit-taking that finds its most famous expression in the work of Karl Marx. It is maintained by proponents of this objection that, as a matter of necessity, if one person gains in some commercial transaction, then this can only have occurred because some other party to the transaction has lost something (Child, 1998, pp. 243–282). *Ex hypothesi* since commercial gain can only arise through some kind of loss; there can never be two beneficiaries in such exchanges. If we hold the zero-sum view of profit, then commercialisation will always involve exploitation.

A third common objection focusses on the effects of commercialisation upon the goods provided. It is claimed by many critics that commercialising affects the nature of the goods produced. How might this be possible? The idea is that the market is not simply a neutral device for allocating goods but in fact it often leads to changes in the quality of the goods. The idea would be that in order to make a profit, commercial medical providers will find the cheapest way of producing the good or service and in this way often do so through the use of inferior materials or less thorough procedures.

A fourth objection concerns the *very meaning* of medicine. The idea is that commercialisation is at odds with the meanings *constitutive* of medicine: healing sick people is the constitutive end of medicine, and hence commercial medicine necessarily violates the proper ends of medicine. This line is pursued vigorously by Bernard Williams in "The Idea of Equality". While addressing the issue of how medical goods should be distributed, Williams (1973, pp. 230–249) defends this idea. Williams argues that if we set preventative medicine to one side, the proper ground of distribution of medical care is ill health. This, he writes, is a necessary truth. However, in many societies, while ill health may work as a necessary condition for receiving medical treatment, 'it does not work as a sufficient condition since treatment costs money, and not all who are ill have the money' (Williams, 1973, p. 240). Hence the possession of sufficient money becomes an additional necessary condition if we are to receive the required treatment, and this Williams finds morally abhorrent. Williams argues that need is the proper ground of treatment. Clearly the suggestion that it is necessarily true that medical resources should be allocated to those in ill health is intimately related, if not identical, to the claim that curing the sick is the necessary aim or end of medical practice.

The fifth and final objection I consider is the so-called 'Commodification Objection', in which concerns are raised about the shift in attitudes brought about by commercialising human organs.[5] The key idea is that commercialising leads us to regard the commercialised objects as mere commodities and, accordingly when applied to the case of medicine, commercialisation would lead medical professionals to regard patients as *mere commodities*. The thought is that the market norms and the proper ideals of medical professionals are mutually exclusive. It is this objection that I wish to explore in more detail herein.

In the next section, I consider a Kantian explication of the commodification objection that focusses primarily on commodification rather than all elements of what commercialisation, as defined herein, entails.

Before exploring the Kantian objection in greater detail, however, it is worth acknowledging the possibility that there could be instances where commercialisation has positive effects upon the moral characters of commercial agents. Certainly Adam Smith thought that this was true, noting in the *Wealth of Nations* that the Dutch being the most commercial are the most punctual. This is a version of what Albert Hirschman (1977, pp. 56–53) labels the '*doux commerce* Thesis' according to which engagement with markets civilises the general population. This might well be true in some circumstances, although I am somewhat sceptical of how extensive those beneficial effects might be. However, be that as it may, the point of this chapter is to identify ways in which commercialisation can corrode commitment to valuable ideals and how we might avoid such corrosion. The fact – if it is a fact – that commercialisation might have additional positive side-effects does not in itself show that concerns with corrosion are not genuine, or that we do not need to find ways to mitigate the undesirable side effects.

4. Explicating the commodification objection in Kantian terms

What reasons might there be for believing that commercialisation leads those commercialising to regard the goods as *mere* commodities? The first point to make here is that the commodificatory attitude is not simply a matter of transforming a good into a commodity. Commodification itself is typically understood as the process of transforming a good with use-value alone – to use Aristotle's terminology – into a good with both use- and exchange-value. This definition has no normative content built into it. A commodificatory attitude, on the other hand, involves treating the thing as a *mere means*, as a mere instrument for the realisation of an agent's goals. But this still is under-described, for there is presumably nothing wrong with treating a hammer as a mere means. To have a commodificatory attitude towards tools surely is unproblematic. Clearly the focus is on those things that should be regarded as intrinsically valuable. The commodificatory attitude, then, is normatively undesirable for those things that should not be treated as mere commodities. Insofar as healthcare services are connected intimately to something of intrinsic value, namely states of health or wellbeing, then the commodification of healthcare services is undesirable.

What reason, if any, do we have for thinking that commerce *in general* leads to such clearly vicious modes of regard? The standard way of understanding this is as a matter of entailment: the market and intrinsic valuation are thought to be mutually exclusive. Many leading philosophers have endorsed the thought that market institutions *necessarily* destroy non-instrumental value, and hence the market and the realm of intrinsic worth are mutually exclusive.

This thesis that market institutions, by setting a price, destroy non-instrumental value, has exerted considerable influence in applied ethics.[6] The most influential discussion of the idea (which I suggest lies at the heart of the Commodification Objection) is to be found in the work of Immanuel Kant. Although there is some debate as to whether Kant intended his thoughts on the relationship between price and dignity to be employed in general debates over the proper range of the market (Gerrand, 1999, pp. 59–67), his work is nonetheless routinely used in applied ethics to draw conclusions about the moral impermissibility of certain forms of commodification.

The distinction between price and dignity appears in the *Groundwork* in the midst of Kant's discussion of the radical difference between 'things' and 'persons'.

Kant argues that 'things' have only *relative* value; they are valuable in so far as someone happens to desire them, in so far as they are useful for some other ends. Persons, on the other hand, are ends-in-themselves and possess a worthiness or dignity (Paton, 1946, p. 188). For Kant, to treat a person with dignity is synonymous with treating her as an end. The value of a person, unlike that of a thing, is unconditional, incomparable and incalculable: persons should not have a price – that is, a value in exchange – for things with a price are substitutable (Petratos, 2018). Price violates the incomparability of persons since price admits to an equivalence. Kant's dictum clearly has implications for discussions about the proper range of the market, for in persons we have beings that *by their very nature* should not be bought and sold (Kant, 1996, p. 177).

Kant's price-dignity dictum can plausibly be regarded as a version of a more general claim about the destruction of value in market contexts, and more specifically the destruction of things that should be intrinsically valued. Let us call this the 'Entailment Thesis', that reads as follows:

(ET) Necessarily if something has a price then it is not intrinsically valued.

It should be noted that, given its formulation as a universal generalisation, if a *single* case can be identified where both price and intrinsic valuation co-exist, then the Entailment Thesis is false.

What mechanisms associated with markets might lead to this destruction of value? How might it do so *necessarily*?

One might plausibly explain the destruction or evacuation of value in terms of the *equivalence* and *substitutability* that market price enables. Universal scales of equivalence come into being with commercial markets. Price equips us with a precise system of calibration for comparing and ranking goods and, thus, in charging a price, we incorporate the commodified good into a system of reckoning in which all goods contained therein are comparable and ultimately replaceable (Simmel, 1991, pp. 92–93).[7] If an activity or entity has a price, then another thing of equivalent monetary value can be put in its stead. *Ex hypothesi*, commodity goods are substitutable, since in the market anything of equivalent monetary value is of equivalent value. Following this line of interpretation, it is the *substitutability* associated with market institutions that is morally salient. Thus, to commodify is to deny the uniqueness and hence the dignity of the commodified good. One might also explain the value-destroying features of price in relation to the claim that commodifying a good involves regarding that good as a tool or mere means for obtaining wealth (Hill, 1992, p. 247).[8] If one offers an item for sale, then *ex hypothesi* one treats that thing as a means to the acquisition of money. Price is conceived of as an expression of the seller's instrumental regard for the thing offered for sale. So in treating a medical good or service as something that has a price, one expresses an instrumental attitude towards it. It might also be plausibly claimed that there is something about the nature of the pursuit of profit that leads us – mistakenly – to view profit as an end in itself at the expense of the good or service being produced in the name of profit.

5. Compossibility cases and the Corrosion Thesis

In considering this conflation of *commodity* with *mere commodity*, it is instructive to revisit the work of Kant since his treatment of the issue is symptomatic of the general drift of philosophical thinking on this topic. In the *Groundwork*, when Kant asserts that everything has a price or a dignity, he appears to assume that having a price must be the same as having a *mere* price. In other places in his work we find related comments about the instrumentalising role of money and profit-seeking. For instance, when discussing the putative harms of prostitution in the *Lectures on Ethics*, he notes that 'to allow one's person for profit to be used by an other for the satisfaction of sexual desire – to make of oneself an Object of demand – is to dispose over oneself as over a thing and to make of oneself a thing on which another satisfies his appetite, just as he satisfies his hunger upon a steak' (Kant, 1963).

The Entailment Thesis suggests that putting a price on a good *necessarily* leads us to treat the commodified good as a *mere* means. However, by way of counter-example, consider the following case. Consider the activities and the attitudes of the traditional family doctor, at least as we might typically conceive of such a figure. For such a doctor, pursuing wealth is certainly a goal. She is animated by the profit motive. But she would not do anything to make a profit; she is in effect a satisficing agent, instead of a maximising one. Nor is it true that she has an instrumentalist attitude towards her work, for such a doctor is also motivated by a desire to heal. Commercialisation is not *necessarily* destructive of relevant philanthropic motives.

Where does this leave the Entailment Thesis that I suggest underpins the Commodification Objection? Does it provide grounds for rejecting the thesis *in toto*?

In response, I propose a weaker version according to which subordination to the market corrodes, rather than necessarily destroys. In contrast to the Entailment Thesis, let us call the weaker version the 'Corrosion Thesis'.

> *The Entailment Thesis*: If one incorporates x into the market, intrinsic valuation of x will, as a matter of necessity, be destroyed.

> *The Corrosion Thesis*: If one incorporates x into the market there will be a strong *tendency* for x no longer to be valued intrinsically.

According to the Corrosion Thesis, there is a tension between market institutions and intrinsic valuation such that intrinsic valuation tends to be destroyed when the two are in proximity (as it were). Market institutions, such as price, *corrode* our capacity to value goods intrinsically.

The Corrosion Thesis involves an account in which causal factors are understood as providing *predisposing factors* towards an outcome, rather than being fully determining. Market institutions provide predisposing factors towards destruction. Within this account a *single* counter-example is not enough to disprove the central thesis. A single counter-example where market institutions and intrinsic valuation coexist does not demonstrate the falsity of the Corrosion Thesis.[9] Additionally, I also endorse the stronger claim that market institutions *tend to corrode* intrinsic valuation. Of course, it is possible to have predisposing factors for eventualities that rarely occur. But the norms associated with market institutions are not like that. When we commodify goods, commodities *tend* to become mere commodities. If this claim is correct, and if market institutions do provide predisposing factors, then we should be particularly wary of buying and selling anything we regard as intrinsically valuable.

6. The Corrosion Thesis and the ideals of medical professionals

How might the ideals of medical professionals, such as respect for patients or the concern for health, be undermined or corroded by commercialisation? In what sense is there a tension between the ideals outlined earlier and the processes of commercialisation? (Notice here that, given the line in the previous section, we will be talking of tendencies rather than entailments.) There is also the question of how we might provide the moral or conceptual resources such that health professionals are better able to avoid the corrosive effects of commercialisation, and following from that concern, there is a question as to whether the Kantian approach provides the requisite resources.

In understanding the potential corrosion of the ideals, there are two related elements: a) the psychological propensity to regard any commercial practice as merely a means to the realisation of profits; and b) the tendency for concerns with other people to be eliminated from consideration. Within commercial society there is an unfortunate tendency for treating not only as a means but also as *mere* means. To be sure, as we noted earlier, treating as a means is not incompatible – at least from a logical point of view – with also treating as an end. In the example in which a medical practitioner might well pursue profit as one of her professional goals without viewing medicine as an instrument for the accumulation of wealth, the point is that the adoption of commercial motives does not mean *ipso facto* that the commercial agent in question regards such activity as a mere means to money. Indeed, there are many cases where it is clear that a person who is undertaking an activity for financial gain also intrinsically values the activity. The fact that many doctors, for example, do what they do for money need not impinge upon their commitment to and belief in the value of what they do in realising the intrinsic good of states of wellbeing and health in their patients. Nonetheless there is a psychological pull within commercial society for purely instrumental profit-seeking to become the norm. There is also the question of the extent to which patients themselves – when they express their rights using consumerist language – add to the commercial atmosphere of medical activity and healthcare. Such behaviour only adds to the pressure upon medical professionals to act in ways contrary to their espoused ideals.

In relation to the ideals of medical professionals, it is possible to identify two key forms of corrosion. The first is what we might call *distraction*. One possible outcome of immersion in a more commercial context is that the medical professionals involved no longer have ideals – such as respect for persons or the wellbeing of the community – at the forefront of their minds when practicing. The second and more disturbing phenomenon involves the loss or devaluing of other-regarding concerns, such that when conflict arises between some ideal and an opportunity for profit, profit wins. Commercially oriented medical professionals being motivated by financial gain can come to lack the kind of other-regarding concerns that are appropriate to medicine. Where pursuing profit comes into conflict with the philanthropic goals of medicine, then there is a danger that commercial agents will allow their profit-seeking to trump any or many other-regarding considerations. Thus, instead of assisting needy people, a commercial medical practitioner might only assist needy people if it is of financial benefit to her. The point is that persons who are motivated by profit can come to lack the requisite other-regarding moral concerns. The profit motive pushes out philanthropic motives from the agent's motivational set, and thus when the occasion arises that the commercial and the philanthropic are in some considerable conflict, philanthropic motives are trumped.

The conclusion, then, is that the presence in commercial medicine of profit motives provides genuine grounds for concern because of two tendencies to which commercial agents, *qua* commercial agents, are prone. There is the tendency for such agents, in cases where significant other-regarding moral considerations clash with economic considerations, to disregard the moral in favour of the economic. There is also the tendency for commercial agents to regard medical practices as a mere means to the acquisition of wealth. The outcomes that ensue from such temptations are at odds with both the general aims of medicine and the proper aims of medical practitioners. In saying this, we should not forget the potential role that patients themselves have to play in both the corrosion of healthcare through consumerist understandings of their rights and, at the same time, to be part of the solution through their rejection of such understandings.

7. Concluding remarks – commercialisation as a moral hazard for health professionals

There are, then, plausible *pro tanto* grounds for rejecting the commercialisation of medicine, some of which were discussed in section 3. Equally, there are also *pro tanto* reasons for defending some forms of commercialisation. Markets function as both incentive and information systems. In the right circumstances, and, in particular, in the absence of monopoly, the incentives that markets provide for producers can encourage innovation and the production of considerable surplus. Markets are capable of generating a superfluity of goods and fostering innovation to an extent so far unachievable in any other social arrangements. Whatever the merits of those competing arguments, commercialisation is likely to continue into the near future. Given that commercialisation continues, then it is important to consider ways of mitigating any possible harm.[10]

One substantial set of social practices that needs to be safeguarded from the threat of corrosion is the ideals of medical professionals. To be sure, there is no apodictic certainty, no necessity about such corrosion: it is not the case that commercialisation will necessarily corrode such ideals. Yet the danger is clear and present. The Corrosion Thesis identifies a phenomenon of real moral significance both generally for any form of commercialisation and more specifically for the ideals of medicine.

Commercialisation then can have morally pernicious effects upon our attitudes, and as such it presents a distinctive *moral hazard*. The term "moral hazard", as used here, refers to temptations for morally vicious behaviour that – given our natural proclivities – certain processes, institutional frameworks or states of affairs might present to us (Kotowitz, 1987). Here, the moral hazard involves our attitudes or modes of regard towards the intrinsically valuable activity of medicine. Note the slightly idiosyncratic usage of the term at play here. In economics, a moral hazard standardly refers to

> actions of economic agents in maximizing their own utility to the detriment of others in situations where they do not bear the full consequences or equivalently do not enjoy the full benefits of their actions due to uncertainty and incomplete or restricted constraints which prevent the assignment of full damages to the agent responsible.
>
> (Kotowitz, 1987, pp. 549–550)

In the present case, by way of contrast, I employ the term 'moral hazard' to cover instances where an institution or practice provides a context in which we become significantly more likely to engage in some vicious action or adopt a vicious mode of regard. The point is not that our dealings with markets are in and of themselves morally wrong, but rather that they involve a context in which there is a high likelihood that we will engage in vicious behaviour and, as such, from a public policy point of view, this implies that some forms of mitigation are required. In this case it would involve the adoption of a vicious mode of regard.

What practical implications might this have? What might it mean for health policy markers who, within a largely commercial context, wish to avoid potential dangers including the corrosion of the ideals of medical practitioners? The response to possible corrosion should be two-fold. First, legislation should be established – if it is not already in place – to restrain and constrain the possibilities of behaviour where the pursuit of profit overshadows significant moral values. Second, medical professionals should be warned of the dangers of regarding medicine as an instrumental activity, and such warnings should be built into professional directives, most notably codes of ethics. While it is permissible to regard the production of cars, for instance, as a mere means, so long as certain other-regarding moral considerations are observed, this is not the case in medicine. Third, there is a need for medical professionals themselves to develop the moral resources (virtues if you like) that would enable them to resist the temptations for vice that commercialisation often places in their way. Space here does not permit an adequate discussion of how professionals might develop and enhance their virtue, but clearly it will also have a role to play in preventing corrosion. Such ideas are explored in considerable detail in the next chapter in this volume (Misselbrook, 2018).

There is a need for both adequate government regulation and vigilance on the part of individual agents, for without these constraints there is a danger that commercial medicine will degenerate into an activity of pure profit-seeking. Here moral philosophy clearly has a place; for in explicitly articulating how commercial medicine might be corrupting, it has a role to play in helping to avoid any excesses of markets, in what is an essential area of human endeavour.

Notes

1 In this chapter, I shall treat 'commercialisation' as the more general term that includes all three of these changes to the systems of production and distribution. Thus 'commodification' is but one element of the broader process of commercialisation.
2 In *Spheres of Justice,* Walzer argues that although commerce has an important and legitimate place in any reasonable society, it should be excluded from certain spheres of activity. He lists 14 examples of what he calls 'blocked exchanges', which are goods that we should not buy and sell.
3 For a sceptical take on the commitment of health services to such ideals, see Miran Epstein's chapter 'The corruption of medical morality under advanced capitalism' in this volume.
4 For a more radical discussion of the exploitation involved in healthcare, see Miran Epstein's chapter in this volume.
5 This term is credited to Stephen Wilkinson in *Bodies for Sale: Ethics and Exploitation in the Human Body Trade* (London: Routledge, 2003). Of course, there are lots of different objections to commodification, but Wilkinson uses the term to refer to this concern with our attitudes towards, and treatment of, commodified goods, and this usage has since become commonplace.
6 It is worth noting that this debate about the role of prices is orthogonal to the debate over the efficiency of pricing as a system for the provision of information, as discussed in Pythagoras Petratos' chapter in this volume. The question here does not concern whether the use of prices is efficient, but whether or not the ascription of prices damages something of intrinsic value.
7 Georg Simmel claims in the *Philosophy of Money* that value arises only through such comparisons – it is price which gives rise to value.
8 Thomas Hill explicates the undesirability of equivalence in terms of instrumental regard.
9 Nor would logically possible, but physically impossible, counter-examples disprove the Corrosion Thesis.
10 Note that I am not adjudicating here on whether or not commercialisation should occur. The question is a conditional one; if commercialisation proceeds then how should we act so as to protect important features of social life, including the proper ideals of medical professionals?

References

Child, J.W. (1998). "Profit: The Concept and Its Moral Features", *Social Philosophy and Policy*, vol. 15, pp. 243–82.
Declaration of Geneva (1948). Adopted by the General Assembly of World Medical Association at Geneva Switzerland, September 1948.
Declaration of Helsinki (1964). Adopted by the 18th WMA General Assembly, Helsinki, Finland, June 1964.

Epstein, M. (2018) "The corruption of medical morality under advanced capitalism", In T. Feiler, J. Hordern, and A. Papanikitas (eds.), *Marketisation, Ethics and Healthcare: Policy, Practice and Moral Formation*, Abingdon: Routledge, pp. 32–49.

Gerrand, N. (1999). "The Misuse of Kant in the Debate about a Market for Human Body Parts", *Journal of Applied Philosophy*, vol. 16, no. 1, pp. 59–67.

Hill, T., Jr. (1992). *Dignity and Practical Reason*, Ithaca: Cornell University Press.

Hirschman, A.O. (1977). *The Passions and the Interests: Political Arguments for Capitalism before Its Triumph*, Princeton: Princeton University Press.

Kant, I. (1963). *Lectures on Ethics*, trans. L. Infield, New York: Harper and Row.

Kant, I. (1996). *The Metaphysics of Morals*, trans. M. Mcgregor, Cambridge, England: Cambridge University Press, pp. 184–6.

Kotowitz, Y. (1987). "Moral Hazards", in J. Eatwell, M. Milgate, and P. Newman, (eds.), *The New Palgrave Dictionary of Economics*, London: Macmillan.

Medical Board of Australia (2014). Good Medical Practice: A Code of Conduct for Doctors in Australia, Canberra.

Misselbrook, D. (2018) "The Virtuous Professional and the Marketplace", In T. Feiler, J. Hordern, and A. Papanikitas (eds.), *Marketisation, Ethics and Healthcare: Policy, Practice and Moral Formation*, Abingdon: Routledge, pp. 147–162

Paton, H.J. (1946). *The Moral Law or Kant's Groundwork of the Metaphysics of Morals*, London: Hutchinson.

Petratos, P. (2018). Why the Economic Calculation Debate Matters: The Case for Decentralisation in Healthcare. In T. Feiler, J. Hordern and A. Papanikitas (eds.), *Marketisation, Ethics and Healthcare: Policy, Practice and Moral Formation*, Abingdon: Routledge, pp. 13–31

Radin, M.J. (1996). *Contested Commodities*, Cambridge, MA: Harvard University Press, pp. 102–4.

Simmel, G. (1991). *The Philosophy of Money*, 2nd enlarged edition, ed. D. Frisby, trans. T. Bottomore and D. Frisby, London: Routledge.

Walsh, A. (2001). "Are Market Norms and Intrinsic Valuation Mutually Exclusive", *Australasian Journal of Philosophy*, vol. 79, no. 4, December, pp. 525–43.

Walzer, M. (1983). *Spheres of Justice: A Defense of Pluralism and Equality*, New York: Basic Books.

Wilkinson, S. (2003). *Bodies for Sale: Ethics and Exploitation in the Human Body Trade*, London: Routledge.

Williams, B. (1973). "The Idea of Equality", in *Problems of the Self*, Cambridge: Cambridge University Press.

9   The virtuous professional and the marketplace

David Misselbrook

Chapter summary

What does it mean to be a virtuous professional? This chapter argues that health-care workers' communities of practice draw their culture both from moral theory and from the marketplace. The chapter explores how healthcare constructs itself as a professional (as opposed to a solely technical or commercial) activity. It explores the role of moral theory (as opposed to instrumental ethical rules) within the practice of medicine.

Market forces are most commonly located within a contractarian moral anti-realist framework (although this is not the case for Nozick's audacious but restricted vision). Whilst deeper moral realist commitments continue to bind much of society together, in the last three decades one particular part of the capitalist narrative – market forces – has increasingly dominated Western culture. In this chapter I argue that whilst classic market theory claims to maximise efficiency of production and distribution of services, it is ill-suited to these tasks within a healthcare context. Current trends in healthcare management seek to give precedence to markets, putting stress on the previous adaptive balance between virtue and market forces.

I argue that if healthcare is to pursue the proper goals of medicine, this turn is morally problematic. Notions of human flourishing which give particular priority to the weak and vulnerable are ill-adapted to a market narrative that sees no problem in the strong dominating the weak.

This chapter examines the moral and professional dilemma caused by this philosophical conflict. I argue that the virtuous practitioner will pursue the *telos* of medicine rather than market forces. This *telos* will be motivated by compassion and implemented by wise means, whilst paying attention to the *polis* or social environment of healthcare, as well as the possible excellences of practitioners.

1. Medical professionalism

Healthcare has lived within its own slowly evolving but clearly located subculture for some two and a half millennia. The Hippocratic tradition's fundamental sympathies lie in a virtue ethic within which recent theories of professionalism are increasingly and frequently nested. Contemporary professionalism is often instrumentalised via a duty-based narrative, however its moral underpinning would not be unfamiliar to Hippocrates in seeing the proper flourishing of the healthcare worker to lie in their attention to the flourishing of others. We can demonstrate this by mapping across the Hippocratic Oath to the UK GMC Good Medical Practice (GMC, 2013). The GMC guidance on the priority of the needs of the patient, good clinical care, working within competence, teaching and training, relationships with patients, working with colleagues and probity all mirror the concerns of the Oath. Only maintaining good medical practice and declarations concerning one's own health are omitted from the Oath, perhaps unsurprisingly in an age when medical knowledge changed slowly and the Hepatitis B vaccination had not been invented. The fact that there is a common thread from Hippocrates to the GMC supports the view that healthcare gives an example of a response to a universal moral duty to help our fellows. This theme will be expanded later in the chapter.

Doctors have traditionally seen themselves as part of a covenant relationship with society (Crawshaw et al., 1995, p. 1553; Cassel, 1996, p. 604). Doctors come from the highest group for academic attainment. They should therefore be able to compete in many highly paid job markets. They undergo a rigorous 5-year undergraduate education followed by 5–9 years of higher training before they can compete for senior posts. Typically, if full time, they work for 50–80 hours/ week (sometimes more), including unsocial hours. They are expected to "make the care of their patients their first concern", to perform to high professional standards, to take responsibility for their own CPD and to have high levels of probity (GMC, 2013).

In return doctors have in the past expected certain benefits from society. These include social standing and respect, professional freedom and self-regulation, good pay (although not the stratospheric pay of the new rich) and a good pension guaranteeing a comfortable retirement. Whilst it is debatable to what extent society's side of the covenant remains, it would be hard to argue that being a doctor does not remain a respected and well-paid job.

However, medical professionalism has other possible interpretations. George Bernard Shaw (1911) stated that "all professions are conspiracies against the laity". Eliot Freidson (1970) saw the professional image of medicine as masking the realities of medicine's dominance of the sick and vulnerable via our exclusive license to diagnose, prescribe and refer.

Foucault (1963, p. 89) accuses the medical tribe of dominating patients rather than sharing power. Via the "the medical gaze" doctors transform the patient's story, fitting it into a biomedical paradigm, filtering out non-biomedical material and thus marginalising the lived illness experience of the patient. For Foucault, medicine creates an abusive power structure.

So does "medical professionalism" represent altruism or avarice? Surely, despite ambivalence, it is usually a bit of both? There is no fundamental moral or cultural problem in the construction of a profession that contains elements of two different cultures. In this instance, the professional virtues of caring can flourish within the broader market driven society which ensures an expert care giver gets appropriately rewarded. One could use Aristotle's methodology of the *golden mean* to define a healthcare profession that finds a well-judged intermediate place between unrealistic altruistic purity and an avaricious monopoly. However, if either culture seeks imperialistically to take possession of the moral domain of the other then fundamental problems arise.

Moral theory is strongly interpreted through, and mediated by, subcultures within any particular society. If we accept a model of a medical professionalism in a healthy and dynamic tension between altruism and market forces, then how is such a balance constructed and maintained? Surely it must be by means of appropriate discourses. Let us then examine the conceptual basis of these discourses.

2. The proper goals for medicine

If I have a clear goal I can work out the best way to get there. So – what are the proper goals for medicine? I have examined this issue elsewhere (Misselbrook, 2015). If we accept that healthcare should aim to maximise health, then what definition of health will be our yardstick? First, I must draw a distinction between three distinct concepts. Disease is a medical model centring on pathology. Illness is the patient's subjective experience of ill health. Disability describes reduced functioning within the external world. These differing concepts leave us with two possible operational definitions of health; the biomedical and the functional.

In the paper cited (Misselbrook, 2015, p. 548), I argued that the proper goal of healthcare should be to "aim for the state of least possible illness or disability, or of maximal functional adaptation to illness or disability". You will notice that this goal contains no reference to disease. Disease is the doctor's territory. Disease only matters instrumentally because it may underlie illness or disability. Our goals for healthcare should relate to real-world outcomes for the patient, not biomedical outcomes for the doctor. Medicine, by minimising illness and disability, should serve human flourishing.

3. Culture conflicts in the healthcare world – managerial culture

Clearly, any organisation needs to be managed. In the past, hospitals were managed by a strong hierarchy of doctors with minimal administrative support (typically the Hospital Secretary, who, together with Matron, would pretty much run the place together.) This worked because of the hierarchical nature of the medical profession, with each doctor's work having little oversight other than the variable and unstructured oversight of "the chief". This was economical and often efficient, but patchy, relying on the vision and methods of the senior staff. It was not always effective, sometimes dangerous and had little regard for the interests of other stakeholders such as other healthcare workers and the patients themselves.

The second half of the twentieth century arguably saw a gradual but purposeful shift towards more patient-centred care (Tuckett et al., 1985). Thus, hopefully doctors and patients were negotiating a more equal relationship, initially with a small management element still tacked on. But according to Himmelstein and

Woolhandler (2003), there has been a 3,000% increase in the number of healthcare managers in the U.S. since 1970, compared with an approximately 160% increase in the number of doctors. (The U.S. population increased by about 50% during this time.) But just as significant as this staggering growth in numbers, is the new *dominance* of management culture.

This is seen not only in the way that healthcare is run but also in the practice of medicine itself. Thus, in the UK we have external management standards imposed, rather than internal standards developed. In England, we have bodies such as the Care Quality Commission (CQC), Clinical Commissioning Groups (CCGs) and NHS England (NHSE) dictating the management structures within which healthcare is run. This may distort local priorities. The paperwork and doctors' time involved takes huge resources away from patient care. But on top of this, the practice of medicine itself is *de facto* dictated by NICE guidelines and, in general practice, Quality Outcome Framework (QOF) requirements. These have only modest effects (if any) on improving biomedical aspects of care (Hippisley-Cox, Vinogradova and Coupland, 2007; Gillam and Siriwardena, 2011). However, they degrade doctors' professionalism and reduce the potential for patient-centred care (Heath, Hippisley-Cox and Smeeth, 2007; Checkland and Harrison, 2010; Grant et al., 2009; Misselbrook, 2011).

Managerial culture differs from doctors' professional culture. Enteman (1993) sees managerial culture as a separation of decision-making from the actual context of work. Whilst increasing accountability, it also entrenches asymmetrical power relationships and hierarchy. Locke and Spender (2011) argue that managerial culture systematically disempowers actual workers throughout whole organisations. In an ironic mirroring of Foucault, Klikauer (2015, p. 1105) argues that:

> Managerialism combines management knowledge and ideology to establish itself systemically in organisations and society while depriving owners, employees . . . and civil society . . . of all decision-making powers. Managerialism justifies the application of managerial techniques to all areas of society on the grounds of superior ideology, expert training, and the exclusive possession of managerial knowledge necessary to efficiently run corporations and societies.

The fundamental idea is one that would have puzzled our forebearers – that within a system of production (as opposed to the governance of a society) the immediate operational decisions should be separated from those carrying out the work and be made, via paper- (or IT-) based models, by those who have no experience or skill in the work itself.

This represents a clash of cultures, not with a new balance of equals in tension, but with a managerial culture imperialistically taking over medical territory. This may well be an affront to doctors' sense of professionalism, but perhaps its moral significance might be confined to the possibility of negative effects on doctors' performance, recruitment and retention. The real moral question is whether managerial culture aligns more or less closely with the proper goals of medicine.

This is not straightforward. One would first have to define: which medicine? The recent historical cultures of medicine in the West vary significantly between the UK, continental Europe and the U.S. The UK NHS philosophy is one of social solidarity. Any UK resident, whether citizen or not, whether a taxpayer or not, is eligible for the full range of available healthcare based on clinical need, not on the ability to pay, and "free at the point of delivery" (NHS, 2011). Social solidarity is an important political concept but is not tied to any one moral theory (although it is often superficially identified as part of political theories within the sphere of socialism, there is no logical necessity to define it within this context). Of course, healthcare always has to be paid for – in the UK this is via central taxation which is not hypothecated. (This is despite the "purchaser/provider split" and the creation of an internal market by the National Health Service and Community Care Act 1990.) According to the Commonwealth Fund Report (2014, p. 2), UK healthcare is the most effective and efficient (and U.S. the least) but is not always patient-centred.

I have argued that the proper goal of healthcare relates to human flourishing, and thus to patient models of illness and disability, not primarily to doctors' biomedical models. Biomedicine is "our" language, to be used instrumentally for benefit in the patient's world. This is where we see that managerial culture does not give us the best means to these goals. Managerial culture may help us within limited parts of the whole project (for example central procurement of supplies), but is a poor match for our overall goals as it seeks to optimise centrally defined biomedical goals, not human flourishing.

Second though, does managerial culture nurture or inhibit moral behaviour? According to MacIntyre (1981, p. 195), moral practices need institutions that sustain them. Managerialism is based on external transactions. Morality is based on motivation by internal excellences. Consider Donabedian's classic medical managerial model (Donabedian, 1966): "structure, process and outcome". First, the structure of the doctor/patient covenant is relational, not primarily contractual. Second, the "managerial gaze" is an industrial process gaze. But the doctor's *goal* is bespoke, not industrial. Third, what outcomes are visible through a managerial gaze? In terms of health gain, they will likely be biomedical, but these are only ever intermediate outcomes with respect to the proper goals of medicine.

MacIntyre (1981, p. 86) comments that the rise of managerialism

> has two sides to it: there is the aspiration to value neutrality and the claim to manipulative power. Both of these, we can now perceive, derive from the history of the way in which the realm of fact and the realm of value were distinguished by the philosophers of the seventeenth and eighteenth centuries. Twentieth-century social life turns out in key part to be the concrete and dramatic re-enactment of eighteenth century philosophy.

Managerialism within healthcare is therefore a moral issue, not merely a cultural issue. I am not arguing that healthcare should not be managed – clearly it should. I am arguing that there are moral reasons why the *culture* of healthcare should be a culture of social solidarity.

4. Markets and morals

We tend to see free markets as a touchstone of capitalism. It is worth remembering that Adam Smith's attraction to free markets was that he saw them as the most efficient instrument for producing wealth and freedom for populations. Smith (1776, p. 329) stated: "In general, if any branch of trade, or any division of labour, be advantageous to the public, the freer and more general the competition, it will always be the more so". Smith's view of capitalism, whilst at ease with earned wealth, was expected to lead to "universal opulence" rather than the winner takes all of a game of Monopoly. He believed, to use the modern phrase, that a rising tide would lift all boats – so called "trickle down" economics. However, evidence over the last century does not support this view. Indeed, there is a fair amount of evidence to the contrary.

Free markets are supposed to be a way of both maximising and balancing the supply of goods via revenue flow. They are therefore one rational way of producing and distributing goods between autonomous and independent agents. In a capitalist model, a producer's motivation for making a product is legitimate profit – as Smith (1776) said: "It is not from the benevolence of the butcher, the brewer, or the baker that we expect our dinner, but from their regard to their own self-interest". In providing healthcare we are clearly providing goods, in the most general sense. So are the goods provided by healthcare the sort of goods that can best be modelled as discreet physical *products*, like pins and grapes, or services such as banking?

Milbank and Pabst (2016, p. 4) helpfully argue that:

> A moral stance does not ask, first of all, what should I do faced with such and such a predicament, but rather what I should consistently be doing at all. What sort of shape should my entire life appropriately take? What sort of character do I want to be and how should I order this desire in an acceptable way to my relationship with others? And those questions . . . can only be answered if we also ask what sort of society all of us want.

I have argued that the purpose of healthcare is to maximise health. I am arguing that, as health is a fundamental good for humans, to maximise this where a need arises becomes a moral goal, as it is directed towards seeking the good of another.

The purpose of markets however is to manage the production and distribution of goods (of which healthcare is certainly an example) via the economic mechanisms and within the systems of justice in question. According to classic free market theory, this should be to overall benefit, but even if we were to accept this at face value we face two problems. There is a lack of evidence of near universal benefit from free markets in general. Benefits tend to favour the rich. But second, we have a greater problem. Free markets work between rational free producers who exchange their goods. Healthcare is needed most by those who are disadvantaged as producers by reason of sickness (particularly chronic disease) or disability. All the evidence from health inequalities suggests that this group also tends to be the poorest (Marmot, 2005). So we have an asymmetry between healthcare need and the ability to produce. This does not matter in a Nozickian society that has no problem with winners and losers, but it becomes a matter of central concern in a Rawlsian society that seeks to moderate accumulation of goods by the few (Nozick, 1974; Rawls, 1971). In most actual economies, it is seen to matter to a greater or lesser extent. If within healthcare we are committed to maximising human health, then there we have a reason to favour Rawls' "difference principle" over Nozick's *laisse faire* approach.

There is therefore a strong moral case both to prefer a social solidarity model over a market model, and a bespoke human flourishing model over a managerial model, for the provision of healthcare. To accept a healthcare model driven by markets, rather than patient need, is to be indifferent to the "corrosion of ideals" described by Adrian Walsh in Chapter 8 above. But corrosion comes easily. Pinsent (2012, p. 108) comments that "it seems particularly easy in human relationships for second-person relatedness to collapse, almost without noticing, into a mere exchange of goods".

So must we accept libertarian capitalism as a sacred given? It is easy enough to defend some form of capitalism on pragmatic grounds – the Utopian alternatives so far seem to end in tears. But we are still left with two basic issues. First, capitalism is a contingent human system, *not* an unchangeable law of nature. Therefore, we have to ask, if we opt for capitalism on pragmatic grounds, what *variety* of capitalism shall we choose? Is free market capitalism the only legitimate social theory?

Yet money has no independent existence within the world. Broadly, it represents labour plus skill. However, money is hardly directly proportional to the sum of both, it also depends on luck plus its own tendency to accumulate. Economists such as Amartya Sen (2010) have widened the gaze of economic theory from seeing only flows of money, goods and services to include issues of welfare also.

We deal with our families through networks of relationships based on commitment, not commerce. There is a deeper principle. We ourselves are not commercial goods. Martin Buber (1923) sees our relations with others not only as an issue of our duty to respect persons, but as an issue of our own transformation as we recognise the humanity in the other. In relating to others, we ourselves are made truly human. The 'I' of 'I – Thou' is different from the 'I' of 'I – It'. 'A person makes his appearance by entering into relation with other persons' To treat another as merely a means to an end is to treat them as an It, not a Thou. In doing so we wrong not only them but ourselves. Pinsent (2012, p. 100) argues that second-person relatedness is a foundational requirement for the existence of virtue.

So is healthcare provision more properly compared to a butcher selling meat or to a parent caring for their child? Whilst it may be closer to a family, properly it is neither. It is something else that shares some common characteristics with both, but it is best described within its own parameters. Healthcare properly exists within a space of social solidarity, not social competition. Its internal relationships are more analogous to the covenant relationships within a family than the contractual and competitive relationships of the marketplace.

5. Virtue reborn?

So if we agree that morals should trump markets in healthcare then what sort of moral theory fits our case? Aristotle was well aware of the different cultural strands within his society, each with their own intuitive ethic. He therefore sought to ground morality itself in a unified and deeper way that did not rely on the culture of any particular social group. Whilst much has been written on virtue ethics in the last few decades, I will ground this chapter primarily in Aristotle and MacIntyre's accounts.

Aristotle (2000, p. 4) observes that man is a part of the world. Everything in the world has both its place and its own nature. For Aristotle, we have a given nature and a given *telos* or goal, and that is the pursuit of *eudaimonia* or the "good life". In his Nichomachean Ethics, Aristotle (2000, p. 11) defines *eudaimonia* as human flourishing, this being the highest good. This is understood as a much richer and deeper concept than mere pleasure. The person who achieves this rich sense of flourishing is one who embodies "*arete*" or virtue (Aristotle, 2000, p. 28). But there is much more to *arete* than just doing good.

For Aristotle, all human activity aims at some goods, but some goods are more important than others. Aristotle saw the highest human good as more than pleasure, fame or material possessions, but rather as a life lived by reason in accord with excellence of character, or *arete*. Good actions will stem from "settled dispositions" to act in a way that manifests such inner excellence. MacIntyre (1981, p. 191) defines a virtue as "an acquired human quality the possession and exercise of which tends to enable us to achieve those goods which are internal to practices and the lack of which effectively prevents us from achieving any such goods". Thus, actions are seen as good only inasmuch as they express such human qualities. Virtue ethics argues that the world is too complex to be navigated by rules and algorithms. For Aristotle, a right act is the act, within a given complex context, that will tend to be performed by one who has this excellence of character. For Aristotle, right acts derive from excellence of character, not rules. Moral action must rely on judgement. Wise judgement is founded upon a network of character traits or "settled dispositions" that must work together. So, as Hursthouse (1999, p. 6) points out:

> According to virtue ethics . . . what is wrong with lying, when it is wrong, is not that it is unjust (because it violates someone's 'right to the truth' or their 'right to be treated with respect') but that it is dishonest, and dishonesty is a vice.

Arete depends upon the hypothesis that humans have some common nature by which we can reference human flourishing and thus those human excellences that lead to flourishing. This view was not popular in recent decades, but it is now again being taken more seriously, perhaps as popular existentialist philosophy becomes moderated by neuroscience and empirical psychology.

In our pluralistic and possibly less high-minded society today, some might disagree with Aristotle's conception of the good life. However, this does not have to be a narrow or prescriptive formula. It is simply to observe that certain ways of being lead to personal flourishing and others do not. Most clinicians who deal with addiction problems and personality disorders would tend to agree. If we can identify some sort human flourishing then perhaps we can also identify the excellences or human "virtues" that characterise those people who we find to be flourishing (Kraut, 2007).

For Aristotle *eudaemonia* is achieved not through what we do or what we possess but by who we are. *Arete* can be recognised by character traits that, when taken together (and for Aristotle they must always be taken together) define human excellence. Aristotle identifies two kinds of virtues: moral virtues established via habituation, and intellectual virtues established by learning and reflection (Foot, 1997, p. 164).

Aristotle's primary moral virtues are courage, self-control, generosity, magnificence, self-respect, good temper, friendliness, truthfulness and justice. Aristotle lists moral virtues as main examples, not as a definitive or restrictive list. Thomas Aquinas (1225–74) has a very different account of virtue, based in the Scholastic Christian tradition but with clear reference to Aristotle (Pinsent, 2012, p. 3). Aquinas promoted also the three Christian virtues of faith, hope & love. MacIntyre (1981, pp. 181ff) surveys possible candidate virtues, brilliantly encompassing both Homer's world and the world of Jane Austen. This, of course, alerts us to the cultural context of virtue theory. So does this give virtue theory a fatal anti-realist mere-culture foundational problem?

But this is to ignore Aristotle's rationale for his concept of human excellence. We have to remember that Aristotle saw human excellence as existing on two axes. First, that of the flourishing individual. Second, of their flourishing within, and contributing to, a flourishing *polis*, or society. Within such a framework we can distinguish Pol Pot from Mother Teresa. We *can* distinguish virtues from vices (and we *are* able to identify virtues insincerely held) supporting a realist model of virtue theory so long as virtue is properly located. For Aristotle, morality is never a private matter – it exists within a social setting and thus always has a political relevance. As MacIntyre (1981, p. 229) says,

> my good as a man is one and the same as the good of those others with whom I am bound up in human community. There is no way of my pursuing my good which is necessarily antagonistic to you pursuing yours because the good is neither mine nor yours peculiarly – goods are not private property.

So how do we foster virtue? Settled dispositions are synonymous with character and this are developed by modelling, training and repetition. If we are fortunate our parents will instill excellence into our character. As adults we learn virtue by recognising it in others, by reflection, by copying it then practicing it repeatedly until it becomes internalised. Learning surgery requires some theory and lots of practice. Learning moral reasoning, according to virtue ethics, requires the same but more – we ourselves are in the frame. It is not an academic activity; it is a personal craft.

Anyone who has dealt with the complexity of real life will know that simple rules are inadequate – they simply fail. And whilst duties and consequences are part of any mature moral assessment they cannot be the only moral concern. Virtue ethics seems at present to be our best moral model because it is grounded in a teleology that seeks human flourishing, that therefore assumes there are ways of living that promote flourishing and ways of living that do not. Aristotle's thesis is that humans with a settled disposition to courage, self-control, generosity, magnificence, self-respect, good temper, friendliness, truthfulness and justice, when controlled by practical wisdom, will flourish. They will not always win in life (or in the market) but they will experience a fuller happiness than mere pokes with a hedonic stick. This is because their lives will tend towards a complete and authentic whole, the life that they would rightly seek, and a life that will enable others around to flourish too. It turns the zero-sum game of global Monopoly into a win/win collaboration. Virtue theory provides the "inference to the best explanation" within moral reflection (Lipton, 1991).

6. The doctor's virtues

So what settled dispositions should a good doctor possess? Aristotle's moral virtues are quoted above. His intellectual virtues are science, craft, *phronesis* or practical wisdom, intuitive reason, philosophical wisdom, political science and judgement.

In considering a twenty-first-century doctor's virtues we can assume abilities such as science and craft. I will concentrate on the moral virtues plus *phronesis*. We do not need to bend Aristotle's list of virtues much to fit them to the purpose of human flourishing within our modern medical culture. Although interestingly I would wish to add in three virtues not directly recognised by Aristotle.

There is only one virtue that we need to bend beyond immediate recognition, which is the virtue of magnificence (or sometimes translated as munificence). This has an "if you've got it flaunt it" celebrity ring to it. This is not Aristotle's account of this virtue – he was not in favour of a celebrity culture. In post-Periclean Athens, magnificence refers to the public duty of the rich to improve state infrastructure. Sure, they would be recognised (no Christian humility in the ancient world!) but it is for the good of the *polis*. For this reason, I have replaced "magnificence" with "humanity" as being an appropriate *medical* virtue. But perhaps famous or powerful doctors should remember the virtue of magnificence. A modern lay example would be Bill and Melinda Gates' funding the research to eradicate malaria.

I would argue that the contemporary doctor who is best equipped to act with moral purpose will (broadly following Aristotle) possesses the following settled dispositions:

- *Courage* – to go against the flow (and against guidelines) when patient need or patient advocacy require this.
- *Temperance* – self-control when faced with unreasonable demands by patients, managers or colleagues.

- *Generosity* – going beyond contractual requirements when prompted by compassion combined together with good judgement.
- *Humanity* – communicating well with patients, seeing them as individual humans who are ends in themselves, not as biomedical problems. This also encapsulates Kant's second formulation of his categorical imperative (Kant, 1998, p. 38) to "so act that you use humanity, whether in your own person or in the person of any other, always at the same time as an end, never merely as a means".
- *Self-care* – recognising our limitations and the needs of our own humanity and that of our families.
- *Diligence* – consistently applying high standards of practice.
- *Respectfulness and mutuality* – again this mirrors Kant's first formulation of his categorical imperative (Kant, 1998, p. 31) to: "act only in accordance with that maxim through which you can at the same time will that it become a universal law". To do as we would be done by.
- *Truthfulness* – patients need "someone who loves truth, and is truthful when nothing is at stake, [they] will be all the more truthful when something is at stake".

(Aristotle, 2000, p. 77)

- *Justice* – all doctors need to divide up resources, especially the valuable resource of time, according to a patient's need, not according to how much we like them.

Aristotle has an overall controlling virtue – *phronesis* or practical wisdom. *Phronesis* acts as the conductor of the orchestra, bringing in each virtue as it is needed. As doctors we possess many guidelines, which may well help in straightforward situations. But the real world is too complex to navigate with guidelines alone. *Phronesis* trumps algorithms and rulebooks.

Phronesis seeks the wise course in the patient's best interest. Evidence and guidelines often relate to linear rules ("if A is X then do Z"). The real world presents us with complex situations ("A is approximately X but we do not know if B is currently Y or W, and it seems likely that D and E will influence this situation in ways that may be difficult to predict"). And the moral world is untidy. Different patients have different priorities. "The advantage of using guidelines and algorithms is that they give a reliable answer and tend to be fair. But might we just be giving poor answers, reliably and fairly? Might the better policy be to teach people to think?" (Misselbrook, 2014).

To tailor Aristotle's list for the purpose of the medical practitioner, I would add (partly following Pellegrino):

- *Compassion* – this is a later Christian virtue, added to the Aristotelian virtues by Aquinas (1996) in his reconceptualisation of Aristotelianism, changing it to fit within the framework of Christian theology. Pellegrino (1995) argues that compassion is the prelude for care – for "concern, empathy and consideration of the patient's plight".

- *Integrity* – this is in fact partly assumed by Aristotle in his insistence that character traits can only work jointly – it is no use my being courageous if I lack other virtues; that will not produce good actions. Virtue is consistent because it authentically represents what is inside me. Pellegrino sees this as entailing "intellectual honesty" with patients and colleagues.
- *Trustworthiness* – Pellegrino sees this as "fidelity to trust and promise". This goes beyond diligence, as doctors must be worthy of trust when dealing with what belongs to another, whether it is their cerebellum or their secrets. It thus includes the Hippocratic commitment to confidentiality. They must fulfil the inherent moral commitments of the profession as well as their legal contract to the state or the patient.

Peter Toon has undertaken an extensive analysis of Virtue Theory in General Practice medicine (Toon, 1994, 1999, 2014). Toon maps MacIntyre's "moral confusion" in the context of medical practice. In *A Flourishing Practice?* Toon, like Pellegrino, identifies the primary medical virtue as compassion, and also lists friendship, temperance, integrity and courage among others. Critically again he locates these virtues within the context of the *polis* – in this case flourishing social institutions.

I would cite compassion as a second controlling virtue for the doctor, alongside Aristotle's *phronesis*. Compassion leads to care. This is a Christian and a Hippocratic virtue. The ancient world generally lacked compassion, at least according to its literature. And of course Nietzsche (2013) condemned compassion *because* it was a Christian virtue, fit only for slaves. But if healthcare is not a caring profession it is nothing.

But compassion must be defended against the remorseless pressures of work, emotional overload, technical demand and biomedical imperialism. The Francis Report (2013) gave a thorough and humane analysis of the scandalous deficiencies of care and compassion in the Mid Staffordshire NHS Foundation Trust. But I was disappointed in its conclusions. Having noted problems with guidelines and tick-box care, it seemed to recommend extra layers of guidelines with new tick-boxes to back them up. Peter Toon (2014, p. 104) comments that "The Francis Report does not use the terms virtue and vice; being mostly written by lawyers and managers not used to thinking in terms of virtue ethics, it would have been surprising if it had done so". Surely the Francis Report is a paradigm case of Adrian Walsh's "corrosion of ideals", which should be reversed by virtue theory's rehabilitation into public life.

So how should the virtuous practitioner function within the healthcare marketplace? I would suggest that the virtuous practitioner may need virtue in fulfilling a number of distinct roles.

7. The doctor as citizen

Humans are social beings. In Aristotle's world it is every citizen's duty to attend as much to the *polis* – to society, to the social space – as to their own business (Aristotle, 1981, 2000, pp. 199ff). This finds a partial echo in Kant's "Kingdom of Ends" in his third formulation of his categorical imperative: "to act only so that the will could regard itself as at the same time giving universal law through its maxim"

(Kant, 1998, p. 42). The good citizen not only follows good social practices but seeks to build them across the social space. Doctors are selected from the top 1% of academic achievers. Their training is rigorous and practical, with a requirement to think for themselves and to communicate. If doctors cannot lead within health-care then who can? Healthcare is too important to be left to politicians. Like most complex human practices, it is best understood from the inside. Doctors also have a responsibility to empower patients to speak. Doctors and patients together should create systems of healthcare that meet patient's needs. Politicians and managers ought not to be left to attempt this by themselves.

This requires constant analysis and constructive criticism within the public domain. It requires doctors not to be hoodwinked or overawed by the wealth and power of Pharma, but to speak truthfully and to act with integrity for the benefit of our patients (Goldacre, 2012). It requires doctors to articulate repeatedly the reasons why an alliance of managerial medicine and market forces is not fit for purpose with respect to the proper goals of medicine.

Doctors need to articulate why medicine should be seen within a social solidar-ity or a welfare model. Within this, market forces should be playing only a minor role. If healthcare cannot be shielded from the corrosion of ideals that seems to be an inevitable consequence of our current capitalism, then doctors need to articulate why they should use the models of Sen and Rawls, rather than the models of Smith and Nozick, to modify capitalism. It requires doctors, as "Kantian legislators" within a democratic society, to advocate practical alternatives, both to those in power and within the media-driven *polis*.

8. The doctor as advocate

If doctors are committed to the proper goals of healthcare then they will seek to help patients to live flourishing lives unencumbered by illness and disability. When they see a medical pathway leading away from their patient's flourishing (for example from unwanted effects of guideline driven prescriptions or interventions), they will have the courage to signpost other paths, and to help patients onto the path that most truly reflects their own values and goals.

Doctors have some influence within local healthcare systems. GPs have a fair degree of control over how their practice is run. Consultants still retain rudimen-tary influence within secondary care systems, particularly if they have the courage to go into medical management or become Clinical Directors. But we should not underestimate the challenge. It is hard to function contrary to a culture's norms. And since the Griffiths Report of 1983, managerial culture has inevitably come to dominate UK healthcare.

The virtuous doctor may have to buck the market. A UK GP has significant control over the workings of their practice, even if they do not have much control over their workload or the type of medicine they practice. The virtuous GP will find the well-judged optimal point between profit maximisation and bankruptcy. Doctors are not mendicants, but neither should they be merchants as they run their practices.

For hospital doctors, there will be less control over the way their healthcare provision is run. Here the challenge will be in the allocation of time and the prioritisation of patients. There will be the need to decide on the judicious resistance of targets (such as the Emergency Department "4 hour wait") where these conflict with patient need. There will be the constant demand to mediate between the needs of patients and the demands of managers. The virtuous doctor will also reflect that the demands of their immediate managers actually reflect the *needs* of those managers who are simply the lower end of a chain gang, with the politicians holding the end of the chain. The virtuous doctor will prioritise patients over managers but will also moderate this by acknowledging their own survival needs within management systems.

9. The doctor as practitioner

Markets were supposed to benefit all parties but in practice tend to create winners and losers. Markets in medicine do not lift all boats. But we must also remember that Hippocratic medicine was supposed to be good for both doctors and patients, yet in practice it led to Foucault's medical imperialism. Whatever the system, the virtuous practitioner will act to pursue the proper goals of medicine for their patient.

Doctors have always worked within constraints. A century ago in the UK when medicine existed entirely in the marketplace, most doctors ran Rawlsian businesses, charging the wealthy the full price or more and charging the poor little or nothing.

For the last decade or more, UK-based GPs have had a very explicit "third person" in the consulting room, in their computer systems whose primary purpose seems to have become to enforce the Quality Outcome Framework (QOF). The virtuous doctor will have the courage to defy the QOF and what may replace it. They must struggle to find the wise mid-point between cowardice (attending to an overdue blood pressure or blood monitoring when a patient is overwhelmed by other issues) and recklessness (ignoring QOF to the point of losing 25% of practice income and having to fire the staff.)

As markets increasingly dominate medical practice, the patient's best interest may easily disappear. If UK medicine follows U.S. Health Maintenance Organization- (HMO-) based medicine further down this route, the clinician will increasingly need the formula of compassion plus *phronesis* to navigate the best *realisable* outcomes for the patient. These may not be the best possible outcomes. It is said that politics is the art of the possible. Medicine is increasingly becoming the art of the possible. We need compassion to point us in the right direction, but we also need *phronesis* to tell us which battles can be won and which are best not fought. Our goal normally should be to maximise patient benefit (as defined by the proper goals of medicine) over a professional lifetime.

10. Conclusions

The challenge to doctors from medical markets is not unique. In ancient Rome doctors were often Greek slaves, but within the limits of the system they tried to work within Hippocratic ideals. In modern times, when doctors were relatively free of market constraints, they acted as much in their own interests as that of their patients. They constructed the medical profession to serve both the patient and their own market interests. Now that they are increasingly constrained by markets constructed by others, they bitterly recognise new masters who are unlikely to treat the profession well. So doctors must adapt. The virtuous practitioner will adapt with compassion and *phronesis*, seeking to serve the interest of the patient but realistically acknowledging their own need to flourish as best they can. The wise practitioner will always seek to subvert the zero-sum game on offer and find a win/win collaboration. The medical profession is likely to last as long as the human race itself. It will always adapt. Let us hope that it is always directed by virtuous practitioners.

References

Aquinas, T. (1996) *Summa Theologiae*. Gilby, T. trans. London, Eyre and Spottiswoode, Vol. 18, 1a 2ae, Qs 18–21.

Aristotle. (1981) *The Politics*. Sinclair, T. trans. London, Penguin, Book III.

Aristotle. (2000) *The Nicomachean Ethics*. Oxford, Oxford University Press.

Buber, M. (1923) *I and Thou*. First published in Germany 1923. Smith, R. trans. New York, NY, Scribner, 1937, republished 2000.

Cassel, C. (1996). The Patient-Physician Covenant: An Affirmation of Asklepios. *Annals of Internal Medicine*, 124(6), pp. 604–606

Checkland, K. and Harrison, S. (2010) The Impact of the Quality and Outcomes Framework on Practice Organization and Service Delivery: Summary of Evidence from Two Qualitative Studies. *Qual Prim Care*, 18, pp. 139–146.

Commonwealth Fund Report (2014) www.commonwealthfund.org/publications/press-releases/2014/jun/us-health-system-ranks-last accessed 29/1/17.

Crawshaw, R., Rogers, D., Pellegrino, E., Bulger, R.J., Lundberg, G., Bristow, L.R. et al. (1995) Patient-Physician Covenant. *JAMA*, 273, p. 1553.

Donabedian, A. (1966) Evaluating the Quality of Medical Care. *The Milbank Quarterly*, 83(4), pp 691–729.

Enteman, W. (1993) *Managerialism: The Emergence of a New Ideology*. Madison, WI, University of Wisconsin Press.

Foot, P. (1997) Virtues and vices. In Crisp, R. and Slote, M., Eds. *Virtue Ethics*. Oxford, Oxford University Press. pp. 163–177.

Foucault, M. (1963) *Naisssance de la Clinique*. Paris, Presses Universitaires de France, 1963. (Republished as *The Birth of the Clinic* [1989] London, Routledge.)

Francis, R. (2013) *Report of the Mid Staffordshire NHS Trust Public Enquiry* ("The Francis Report"). London, Her Majesty's Stationary Office.

Freidson, E. (1970) *Profession of Medicine: A Study of the Sociology of Applied Knowledge*. New York, Harper and Row Publishers.

Gillam, S. and Siriwardena, A. (2011) *The Quality and Outcomes Framework*. Oxford, Radcliffe Press.

GMC (2013) *Good Medical Practice*. www.gmc-uk.org/guidance/good_medical_practice/duties_of_a_doctor.asp accessed 11/1/17.

Goldacre, B. (2012) *Bad Pharma: How Medicine Is Broken and How We Can Fix It*. London, Fourth Estate.

Grant, S., Huby, G., Watkins, F., Checkland, K., McDonald, R., Davies, H., and Guthrie, B. (2009) The Impact of Pay-for-Performance on Professional Boundaries in UK General Practice: An Ethnographic Study. *Sociology of Health and Illness*, 31, pp. 229–245.

Heath, I., Hippisley-Cox, J., and Smeeth, L. (2007) Measuring Performance and Missing the Point? *BMJ*, 335, pp. 1075–1076.

Himmelstein, D., and Woolhandler, S. (2003) US Bureau of Labor Statistics, NCHS analysis of CPS.

Hippisley-Cox, J., Vinogradova, Y., and Coupland, C. (2007) *Time Series Analysis for Selected Clinical Indicators from the Quality and Outcomes Framework 2001–2006.* Nottingham, QResearch and the Information Centre for Health and Social Care.

Hursthouse, R. (1999) *On Virtue Ethics.* Oxford, Oxford University Press.

Kant, I. (1998) *Groundwork of the Metaphysics of Morals.* Gregor, M. ed. Cambridge, Cambridge University Press.

Klikauer, T. (2015) What Is Managerialism? *Critical Sociology*, 41(7–8), pp. 1103–1119.

Kraut, R. (2007) *What Is Good and Why: The Ethics of Well-Being.* Cambridge, Harvard University Press.

Lipton, P. (1991) *Inference to the Best Explanation.* London, Routledge.

Locke, R. and Spender, J. (2011) *Confronting Managerialism.* London, Zed Books.

MacIntyre, A. (1981) *After Virtue.* London, Duckworth.

Marmot, M. (2005) Social Determinants of Health Inequalities. *Lancet*, 365, pp 1099–1104.

Milbank, J. and Pabst, A. (2016) *The Politics of Virtue.* London, Rowman and Littlefield.

Misselbrook, D. (2011) The Quality Outcome Framework: A Critical Assessment. Chapter 4 in Wald, N. and Misselbrook, D., Eds. *The Future of Prevention in Cardiovascular Disease.* London, RSM Press. pp. 31–39.

Misselbrook, D. (2014) An A-Z of Medical Philosophy: P Is for Phronesis. *BJGP*, 64(621), p. 191.

Misselbrook, D. (2015) Aristotle, Hume and the Goals of Medicine. *Journal of Evaluation in Clinical Practice*, 22(4), pp. 544–549.

NHS. (2011) *NHS Core Principles.* www.nhs.uk/nhsengland/thenhs/about/pages/nhscore-principles.aspx accessed 29/1/17.

Nietzsche, F. (2013) *The Genealogy of Morals.* London, Penguin Classics.

Nozick, R. (1974) *Anarchy State and Utopia.* New York, Basic Books.

Pellegrino, E. (1995) Toward a Virtue-Based Normative Ethics for the Health Professions. *Kennedy Institute of Ethics Journal*, 5(3), pp. 253–277.

Pinsent, A. (2012) *The Second-Person Perspective in Aquinas' Ethics.* New York, Routledge.

Rawls, J. (1971) *A Theory of Justice.* Cambridge, MA, Harvard University Press.

Sen, A. (2010) Equality of What? in MacMurrin, S. M., *The Tanner Lectures on Human Values*, 4 (2nd ed.), Cambridge, Cambridge University Press, pp. 195–220.

Shaw, G. (1911) *The Doctor's Dilemma* (play), Act 1. London: OBS, 1956.

Smith, A. (1776) *The Wealth of Nations.* Sutherland, K., Ed. Oxford: Oxford University Press 2008.

Toon, P. (1994) *What Is Good General Practice?* London, Royal College of General Practitioners.

Toon, P. (1999) *Towards a Philosophy of General Practice.* London, Royal College of General Practitioners.

Toon, P. (2014) *A Flourishing Practice?* London, Royal College of General Practitioners.

Tuckett, D., Boulton, M., Olson, C., and Williams, W. (1985) *Meetings between Experts: An Approach to Sharing Ideas in Medical Consultations.* London, Routledge.

10 Empathy in healthcare

The limits and scope of empathy in public and private systems

Angeliki Kerasidou and Ruth Horn

Introduction

Healthcare professionals are expected to care for their patients in an empathetic way. In fact, empathy is one of the core values of the medical profession. Empathy is the ability to understand a person's standpoint, their experience of illness and, through this cognitive resonance, feel motivated to help them. Empathetic doctors and nurses can better care for their patients by addressing their worries and concerns and providing the right treatment for them. Numerous studies have demonstrated the beneficial effects of empathy on patient outcomes, establishing its crucial role in the provision of good healthcare (Boker et al. 2004; Marcum 2013; Spiro 1992; Tsao and Yu 2016). It is important, therefore, that empathy is embraced and promoted not only by the profession but also by the healthcare system as a whole. We argue that empathy exercised by the individual healthcare professional alone is not enough to ensure empathetic care overall. Rather, the healthcare system as a whole needs to embrace empathy as one of its principles and make it the basis on which it operates. Although the professional code teaches doctors and nurses to engage empathetically with their patients, it is difficult for healthcare professionals to develop and maintain this value in a system that does not support and foster it. Operating as an individual in a system that does not share and support core professional values makes maintaining and enacting these values challenging.

In this chapter we examine the two dominant healthcare models, public and private, and discuss the extent to which each model can promote empathetic care. We analyse the moral underpinnings of each model and examine the different justifications for the provision of healthcare under each system. In the public system, provision of healthcare is based on the acknowledgement of interdependence built on the notion of solidarity. In the private system, provision of healthcare is based on the ability to pay or on charity for those who cannot pay. This system is built on the idea of individualism. Individualism promotes personal choice and freedom. On the other hand, solidarity denotes interconnectedness and relatedness. These characteristics of solidarity are also crucial for the development of empathy. Ensuring empathetic care for all can be better achieved in a system that acknowledges people's interdependence and mutual responsibilities.

1. Empathy in healthcare

Empathy is a fundamental value of the healthcare profession. Expert knowledge and technical skills are essential for doctors and nurses to care for their patients, but it is also important that care is provided in an empathetic way. Empathy is the process that allows an individual to understand the world from another person's standpoint and to join in someone else's experiences and feelings (Hojat et al. 2001; Hojat et al. 2002). Empathy requires an emotional involvement with the other without, however, assuming their emotional position or projecting one's own emotions onto them. It entails the ability to be attentive to the difference between own and others' feelings, which makes empathy distinct from sympathy. Empathy is the precursor of compassion, as it is empathy that drives the desire to act in order to address someone else's needs (Goetz et al. 2010; Nussbaum 1996). The caring side of healthcare professions demands attention to this skill.

According to Pellegrino, healthcare professionals, by virtue of their role in and its importance to society, should be committed not only to technical expertise and knowledge, but also 'to something other than self-interest when providing their services' (Pellegrino 2002). Unlike a skilled technician, a healthcare professional needs more than just specialist knowledge to provide good care. That is, in order to exercise their profession, doctors and nurses need to feel empathy and be compassionate towards their patients. Healthcare professions embody a particular socio-moral character, expressed through empathy and compassion, which prevents the physician or nurse from viewing their relationship with the patient 'as primarily a commodity transaction, a contract for service or the mere application of scientific knowledge on a sick organism' (Pellegrino 2002).

Competency and empathy are often described as the two pillars of the healthcare profession. If competency is what allows physicians to provide the right diagnosis, prognosis and treatment, empathy is what allows them to care for their patients and understand their needs. According to Zinn, empathetic care not only allows the healthcare professional to understand the situation from the patient's point of view, but also allows the patient to share their concerns and suffering with their doctor or nurse (Zinn 1993). As shown elsewhere (Kerasidou and Horn 2016), empathy is sometimes misrepresented as emotional over-involvement (sympathy) and seen as harmful to the exercise of technically skilled practice. Taking emotions seriously, especially amongst physicians, is often perceived as a sign of weakness or incompetence, or even as being irrelevant to the provision of healthcare. However, a number of studies demonstrate the benefit of a healthcare professional's ability to critically reflect on emotions and their ability to feel empathy. Empathy is associated with increased patient satisfaction, improved adherence to therapy, decreased medical errors, fewer malpractice claims and better health outcomes (Hickson et al. 2002; Riess et al. 2012). On the other hand, studies have suggested that lack of empathy could result in reluctance to seek help even when needed (Wagner et al. 2007). This highlights the interpersonal character of healthcare. It is much harder for a person to trust, seek help and accept treatment from someone who does not seem to compre-hend their situation or care for them. Without empathy as the motivation for and vehicle by which care is delivered, the encounter risks becoming a mere commodity transaction.

Empathy is also important for healthcare professionals' wellbeing. It can help them guard against emotional exhaustion and depression, and deal with emotional distress such as patient suffering, illness and death (Halpern 2003; Kerasidou and Horn 2016). Empathy requires reflection and awareness of one's own emotions and feelings as a way of acquiring and maintaining the appropriate mental and emo-tional resources to deal with the pain and suffering of the people around them. The more people learn to be sensitive and respectful of their own needs and emotions, the more sensitive and respectful they also become of the needs and emotions of others (Wiklund Gustin and Wagner 2013; Raab 2014).

Although empathy is perceived and experienced as a characteristic of the indi-vidual doctor or nurse, the development of empathy as a primary motivator of care cannot be left solely in the hands of the healthcare professionals. This is demonstrated by the great attention medical education gives to the development of empathy (Wald 2015; Dehning et al. 2013; Davis 1990; Boker et al. 2004; Spiro 1992; Marcum 2013). There is a wide recognition that in order for professional values, such as empathy, to be fully developed, the system in which the profession-als operate should also be committed to the promotion of these values. Systems and institutions have their own moral character, and as such they have the ability to promote or constrain the actualisation of particular professional attributes and characteristics (MacIntyre 1985; Titmuss, 1976). Therefore, looking at the way healthcare systems are organised, and the type of values they advocate and pro-mote, is important. In what follows, we will discuss the ability of the two dominant healthcare models, private and public, to accommodate and foster empathy as an essential part of the medical profession. We will first outline how the moral underpinnings of each healthcare system link to empathy, and then discuss how empathy is cultivated and encouraged in each system.

2. The moral underpinnings of the public and the private healthcare models

2.1 *Public healthcare system and solidarity: acknowledging interdependence*

There are different ways to organise healthcare provision. Healthcare can be pro-vided through public funding that is drawn from general taxation or public contri-butions; this is what we call public healthcare provision. Alternatively, healthcare can be organised as a private service that can be purchased at the point of need by the patient; this is what we will call private healthcare provision. These two ways of providing care are not always mutually exclusive, and various combinations of public and private care provision can co-exist within one system. For example, in the UK, the National Health System (NHS), which is funded through general taxation and national insurance contributions, buys many services from private providers, such as psychiatric care and long term residential care (Doyle and Bull 2000). In the U.S., although healthcare facilities are largely operated by private companies, still a large proportion of healthcare expenditure is covered by the state, through insurance programs such as Medicare (Himmelstein and Woolhandler 2016). Also, very often healthcare services are provided by the third-sector, such as charities. However, for the purposes of this chapter, we will talk about public and private healthcare systems, not as a way of reflecting *real* systems, but as a tool to differentiate between the different justifications and moral underpinnings of each healthcare system; one that sees care as a right and a good that should be equally distributed to all members of society (public), and another that understands healthcare as a service to be privately purchased (private). We argue that in a public system, healthcare provision is based on the principle of solidarity, whereas in the private system it is based on the principle of individualism and liberty. These different moral underpinnings influence the way empathy is nurtured in each system.

Publicly funded healthcare systems are premised on the principle that there is a positive right to welfare, including healthcare. This means that people have an obligation to fulfil this right not only by refraining from interfering with one's welfare but by actively promoting it (Buchanan 1987). Daniels justified the positive right to healthcare by arguing that equal access to healthcare is a matter of justice as it protects normal functioning which contributes to protecting equality of opportunity (Daniels et al. 2000). Seeing access to healthcare as a duty of justice means that it can be enforced. Governments around the world have enforced equal access to healthcare to all members of society either through taxation or compulsory contribution to an insurance system. Citizens pay into the common purse according to their means, and the funds are used to distribute healthcare resources to all citizens according to their needs. A system that endorses wealth distribution as a way of addressing the needs of those worse off exhibits the principle of solidarity as it acknowledges the importance of 'mutual respect, personal support and commitment to a common cause' (ter Meulen 2015). The principle of solidarity that underpins the public healthcare system emphasises the interdependency of members of a society and their duties to each other.

Durkheim was the first to develop an account of social solidarity and individuals' interrelatedness with each other. He showed that individualised modern societies that do not depend anymore on strong familial bonds and traditional values maintain their social order by recognising the extent to which each of their members rely on each other (Durkheim 2014). Durkheim called this 'organic solidarity'; the social bond emerging through the recognition of individual needs and of shared duties to address those needs. In the healthcare context, it is this acknowledgement of interdependence and of the importance of social cohesion that creates the moral commitment of a society to accept the equal distribution of goods in order to guarantee equal access to care. Such a moral commitment, or 'collective consciousness' (Durkheim 2014), strengthens the social ties and encourages relatedness to each other (MacIntyre 1985; Durkheim 2012). The public healthcare system is thus based on the moral value of reciprocal responsibility, which reflects a feeling of belonging together and a relationship of mutual support and cooperative practice that aims to a greater good (ter Meulen 2015). As we will develop later, these feelings of responsibility, and recognition of obligations toward all members of society, imply empathy with the conditions of others and a willingness to care (Stjernø 2009, p. 185).

2.2 Private healthcare and individualism: choosing to benefit others (or not)

Private healthcare systems are premised on the ideals of the right to liberty and the right to property. These (and the right to life) are described as natural rights – rights we all possess in virtue of our nature. Natural rights are distinguished from social rights, such as the right to healthcare, which are those imposed by government or society. Social rights can be accepted only as long as they do not infringe upon natural rights. In the case of a universal access to healthcare, ensuring such a right would require wealth redistribution by the state (e.g. general taxation). Yet, general taxation to safeguard a social right in effect violates people's natural rights to liberty (freedom of choice) and property (freedom to enjoy one's fruits of labour). According to Nozick, the state should not impose moral obligations on its citizens, including coercing citizens to donate their resources to assist others. Even if such an obligation would be socially optimising, doing so would be analogous to forced labour (Nozick 2013). Individuals should be allowed to purchase healthcare privately, and thus exercise their right to liberty and property as well as promote their own conception of good. Purchasing healthcare privately promotes individual freedom and ensures appropriate use of resources (Epstein 1997). The principle that underpins the private healthcare system is individualism. Individuals are free to exercise their right to pursue the good life as they see it, without being coerced or constrained by externally imposed moral norms.

An unavoidable consequence of a private system, however, is that some individuals might find themselves in a situation where they cannot afford the appropriate care (e.g. very expensive cancer treatment). In those cases, the only acceptable way for these individuals' needs to be met is through charity. Charity, one's resolve to freely give to others, is the free expression of one's moral code and character.[1] A person can decide to charitably give away their property, or part of it, to another for the other person's benefit (beneficence) in accordance with their own social and moral convictions. The exercise of charity respects both the right to liberty (the giver decides how to use their property) and property (the donation is voluntary), and is consistent with the principle of individualism. A state-enforced charity (e.g. wealth redistribution through taxation) would not only violate natural rights, but would also undermine the nature of charity by making it an enforceable duty, rather than an autonomous expression of free choice and moral character.

The idea of individual freedom of choice defended by the private healthcare system contrasts with the collective aspects of solidarity found in the public healthcare system. The values of individual freedom and possibility of choice challenge the idea of interdependency, mutual responsibility and collective solidarity. The private healthcare system does not foreclose concern and care for those who cannot afford it, but neither does it require it. Its members are not expected to consider their relatedness to each other, as it does not recognise any mutuality or commonality amongst them. Rather, it expects them to operate on the basis of rational self-interest. Even though charity indicates generosity, List argues that it is often construed as connoting "self-sacrifice" (List 2011). The individualistic aspect of charity does not presuppose a shared value system. That is why it leaves the distribution of benefits in the hands of individuals. As we will develop in the following section, the absence of mutual responsibility and recognition of each other's needs does not encourage engagement with other persons' perspectives, which is fundamental for the development of empathy.

3. The impact of different moral underpinnings on empathetic perspective taking

3.1 The scope of empathy in the public healthcare system

We argued above that a public healthcare system is premised on the principle of solidarity, recognises commonality and mutuality, and relies on a symmetric relationship between people. Solidarity shares features with charity in as much as both principles describe one's willingness to bear costs to assist others, 'but they differ importantly with regards to the element of sameness and the type of relationship between giver and receiver' (Prainsack and Buyx 2012). The feeling of belonging together makes it easier to relate to each other and enhances the ability to see the world through the eyes of the other. This process is fundamental for the development and exercise of empathy (Stjernø 2009). Fostering empathy within society facilitates the process of wealth redistribution, which is seen as part of one's social responsibility. The inter-subjectivity and concern for the wellbeing of others provides the moral ground for the public healthcare model.

At this point it is important to emphasise the iterative relationship between developing particular principles and aptitudes at a systemic level and at an individual or professional level. A healthcare system that endorses and promotes a strong empathetic regard for the welfare of others facilitates the exercise of empathy in the delivery of care. Studies have demonstrated that empathy is easier to achieve when it is directed towards people with whom we identify, e.g. people from similar social and educational backgrounds (Stürmer et al. 2005), but not so easy in the absence of a sense of mutuality with the other. As de Waal observes, it is more difficult to be empathetic towards and identify with 'people whom we see as different or belonging to another group' (De Waal 2009). A considerable amount of moral work would be required from the individual to overcome embedded prejudices. Promotion of social cohesion, therefore, becomes crucially important for the provision of empathetic care. A healthcare system that is built on the principles of solidarity and social responsibility encourages relatedness with people from different backgrounds and social groups, and thus promotes social cohesion which facilitates the development of empathy. Empathetic insight and compassionate treatment are part of the requirements of the medical profession. Healthcare professionals ought to deliver empathy and compassion as much as they ought to deliver competent clinical care. Therefore, a solidarity-based healthcare system supports doctors and nurses in the exercise of their professional duties. It trains and educates professionals to develop the norms of reciprocity and care of each other (Stjernø 2009, p. 298). The moral character of the profession aligns with the moral character of the healthcare system, providing a better ground for the exercise and development of empathetic care.

Healthcare systems can play an important normative function by educating professionals to develop norms and moral skills. The normative relationship between the system and the professionals who operate moves both ways. The profession has the ability to influence the way that care is provided, but the ability of the system to foster or constrain special norms should not be underestimated. Titmuss, for example, argues that a healthcare system that recognises everybody's right to care fosters solidarity and social inclusion (Titmuss and Seldon 1968). Buchanan also demonstrates how social institutions and systems can inculcate beliefs and encourage moral behaviour (Buchanan 2002). Pellegrino discusses this in relation to the healthcare profession as a meeting of ethics and *polis*. The values of the social system need to support and nurture the particular values embedded in the healthcare profession (Pellegrino 2002). A solidaristic healthcare system would, therefore, allow empathy in the provision of care to flourish. Furthermore, understanding empathetic care as an expression of solidarity rather than charity underlines the belief that all patients are equally entitled to it.

3.2 The scope of empathy in the private healthcare system

The principles of liberty and individualism that underpins the private healthcare system do not presuppose a moral commitment to common values (other than those of liberty and individualism). Rather, each individual is free to form their own beliefs of what is good. In this way, it neither encourages nor inhibits individuals to, for example, act charitably towards others. In a private healthcare system, there is no expectation to feel social responsibility or to recognise the needs of others. Although the healthcare profession endorses empathy as a core principle, the healthcare system itself remains agnostic towards the need for and importance of empathetic care. This does not mean, however, that healthcare in a private system consistently lacks empathy. Individual doctors and nurses can choose to be empathetic and compassionate towards their patients, even at a cost to themselves. The private system, by allowing individual morality to emerge, creates room for values like charity to function, but it has no interest in promoting this behaviour. In other words, this system does not foster a moral commitment to charity, but leaves it to the individual to decide whether they would like to incorporate it into their own personal moral habitus. Yet, reliance on charity as a way of delivery of care can be problematic. Even the most fervent supporters of a private system admit that it is unlikely that all healthcare needs could be met by relying only on charity

(Epstein 1997). This is a system that is based primarily on self-interest, which does not actively invite people to think about the needs of others. In this way, it refrains from developing social cohesion and a sense of mutuality, which can inhibit the development of empathy.

But how detrimental is the lack of clear moral direction for the delivery of empathetic care in a private system? Consider these two possible ways in which the provision of empathetic care might be impeded in such as system. First, healthcare professionals might fail to develop empathy towards all patients. The private healthcare system is an exclusive system in so far as it offers care only to those who can pay for it. Those who cannot afford to pay for their healthcare are positioned outside the remits of the doctor's or nurse's professional responsibility. A healthcare professional might, therefore, feel less committed towards these patients. One could question, therefore, whether a physician or a nurse who reserves their empathy only for those patients who can pay, can still be said to possess the professional trait of empathy. However, to understand this case just as a failure of the individual to correctly apply empathy and compassion in his everyday dealings would be short-sighted and incomplete, argues Buchanan. This is because such an analysis would ignore the role institutions play in promoting particular behaviour and (mis)guide action (Buchanan 2002). If the healthcare professional decides to treat the non-paying patient out of charity, this would be seen as going beyond the expectations of the system. Such an act would be commendable, especially in situations where caring for such patients can come at a high personal cost for the healthcare professional. Yet, it is questionable for how long individuals could remain charitable in a system that is indifferent to such acts. An individual's moral resources could be quickly depleted, often leading to burnout (Preciado Serrano et al. 2010), or moral aspirations abandoned when operating in challenging conditions. A recent study that investigated the experiences of Greek healthcare professionals working under austerity in a resource-poor and understaffed environment revealed that these challenging conditions impacted on their ability to provide empathetic care. Even though they tried to maintain empathetic care in this adverse environment as best as they could, they expressed their worries and concern about whether they would be able to maintain the 'fight' for long (Kerasidou et al. 2016). Of course, one could point to the continuous existence of healthcare charities as a demonstration that individual heroism is sustainable. Furthermore, it could be argued that those who will be providing healthcare out of charity, and those choosing to work in charitable healthcare institutions, will have a moral attitude and character disposition conducive to empathy and compassion. It is likely, therefore, that empathetic care would be more readily available in a private healthcare system than in a public one. However, the fact that charities are consistently unable to meet the needs of all those who cannot pay for their healthcare proves that relying on charity for empathetic care is ineffective.

Second, an exclusive system does not foster empathy towards those who are marginalised. As Segal describes, lack of empathy and interest in understanding others' situations can lead to blame culture where out-groups are held responsible for their own misfortune (Segal 2011). Glick develops the concept of the 'ideological model of scapegoating'. According to Glick, scapegoating is the result of trying to explain the misfortune of those who are seen as different and unworthy of empathy (Glick 2005; Glick 2002). The unwillingness of an exclusive system to understand other persons' different social, economic and health situations can lead to stereotypes that serve as rationales for the hardship they face. The endorsement of empathy as a professional skill might help doctors and nurses avoid making this type of value judgements for their patients. However, professionals who operate in a system that does not support or encourage the promotion of mutuality between diverse groups might find it difficult to treat 'undeserving' patients the same as 'deserving' ones. They might be less inclined to spend time to counsel, comfort and explain things to 'undeserving' patients, out of concern that their time could be better used caring for those who merit it. As Segal argues, 'empathy that is informed by strong social values such as social responsibility and social justice can overcome stereotyping and blaming of outgroups' (Segal 2011, p. 271). Hence, a system that emphasises interdependence and mutual responsibility could help avoid the stigmatisation and blaming of those who are marginalised.

4. Conclusion

Mutuality and relatedness are fundamental for the development of empathy. Solidaristic systems aim at promoting interrelatedness between people as a way of building social cohesion and supporting acceptance of social responsibilities. A healthcare system that is founded on the principle of solidarity acknowledges the right to healthcare for all on the basis of mutuality and dependency with one another. The acknowledgement of the relatedness with individual patients and the recognition of their perspectives is the prerequisite for empathetic care. In a solidaristic healthcare system, providing appropriate care to everyone becomes a value of the whole system, and not only a value of the profession or of the individual. Under these conditions, it is easier to ensure that empathy is present at the healthcare professional/patient encounter.

On the other hand, a healthcare system that is premised on the principles of liberty and individuality is not concerned with the promotion of a sense of mutuality and social cohesion. It is an exclusive system that provides care only to those who can afford it. For those who cannot afford to pay for their care, charity can fill the space of solidarity. Charitable care, however, relies solely on the motivation of the individual. Charity is not a systemic value or characteristic. Healthcare professionals may still be committed to the provision of empathetic care, yet, maintaining this skill is more difficult in a system committed to other values that do not include charity and empathy. Therefore, if the goal is to provide good care to all, then endorsing a system that is premised on the principle of solidarity rather than one supported by individualism should be preferred.

Note

1 The virtue of charity has its roots in the Christian tradition. Along with faith and hope, it is one of the three theological virtues listed by Aquinas. For Aquinas, charity is a self-perfecting virtue, one that aims at perfecting one's ability to love God, and by extension everything that exists, since God is the master and creator of all.

References

Boker, J. R., Shapiro, J. & Morrison, E. 2004. Teaching empathy to first year medical students: Evaluation of an elective literature and medicine course. *Education for Health*, 17, 73–84.

Buchanan, A. 1987. Justice and Charity. *Ethics*, 97, 558–575.

Buchanan, A. 2002. Social moral epistemology. *Social Philosophy and Policy*, 19, 126–152.

Daniels, N., Kennedy, B., Kawachi, I., Cohen, J. & Rogers, J. 2000. *Is Inequality Bad for Our Health?*, Boston, Beacon Press.

Davis, C. M. 1990. What is empathy, and can empathy be taught? *Physical Therapy*, 70, 707–711.

Dehning, S., Gasperi, S., Krause, D., Meyer, S., Reiss, E., Burger, M., Jacobs, F., Buchheim, A., Mueller, N. & Siebeck, M. 2013. Emotional and cognitive empathy in first-year medical students. *ISRN Psychiatry*, 6. www.hindawi.com/journals/isrn/2013/801530/

De Waal, F. 2009. *Primates and Philosophers: How Morality Evolved*, Princeton, NJ, Princeton University Press.

Doyle, Y. & Bull, A. 2000. Role of private sector in United Kingdom healthcare system. *BMJ: British Medical Journal*, 321, 563.

Durkheim, E. 2012. *Moral Education*, Mineola, New York: Courier Corporation.

Durkheim, E. 2014. *The Division of Labor in Society*, Steven Lukes (ed), New York: Free Press.

Epstein, R. 1997. *Mortal Peril: Our Inalienable Right to Health Care?*, Reading, Mass., Harlow: Addison-Wesley.

Glick, P. 2002. Sacrificial lambs dressed in wolves' clothing. *Understanding Genocide: The Social Psychology of the Holocaust*, L. S. Newman & R. Erber (eds), New York: Oxford University Press, 113–142.

Glick, P. 2005. Choice of scapegoats. *On the Nature of Prejudice*, 50, 244–261.

Goetz, J. L., Keltner, D. & Simon-Thomas, E. 2010. Compassion: An evolutionary analysis and empirical review. *Psychological Bulletin*, 136, 351–374.

Halpern, J. 2003. What is clinical empathy? *Journal of General Internal Medicine*, 18, 670–674.

Hickson, G. B., Federspiel, C. F., Pichert, J. W., Miller, C. S., Gauld-Jaeger, J. & Bost, P. 2002. Patient complaints and malpractice risk. *JAMA*, 287, 2951–2957.

Himmelstein, D. U. & Woolhandler, S. 2016. The current and projected taxpayer shares of US health costs. *American Journal of Public Health*, 106, 449–452.

Hojat, M., Mangione, S., Nasca, T. J., Cohen, M. J., Gonnella, J. S., Erdmann, J. B., Veloski, J. & Magee, M. 2001. The Jefferson scale of physician empathy: Development and preliminary psychometric data. *Educational and Psychological Measurement*, 61, 349–365.

Hojat, M., Gonnella, J. S., Nasca, T. J., Mangione, S., Vergare, M. & Magee, M. 2002. Physician empathy: Definition, components, measurement, and relationship to gender and specialty. *American Journal of Psychiatry*, 159, 1563–1569.

Kerasidou, A. & Horn, R. 2016. Making space for empathy: Supporting doctors in the emotional labour of clinical care. *BMC Medical Ethics*, 17, 8.

Kerasidou, A., Kingori, P. & Legido-Quigley, H. 2016. "You have to keep fighting": Maintaining healthcare services and professionalism on the frontline of austerity in Greece. *International Journal for Equity in Health*, 15, 1–10.

List, J. M. 2011. Beyond charity – social justice and health care. *Virtual Mentor*, 13, 565.

Macintyre, A. 1985. *After Virtue*, London, Duckworth.

Marcum, J. A. 2013. The role of empathy and wisdom in medical practice and pedagogy: Confronting the hidden curriculum. *Journal of Biomedical Education*, 8.

Nozick, R. 2013. *Anarchy, State, and Utopia*, New York: Basic books.

Nussbaum, M. 1996. Compassion: The basic social emotion. *Social Philosophy and Policy*, 13, 27–58.

Pellegrino, E. D. 2002. Professionalism, profession and the virtues of the good physician. *Mt Sinai Journal of Medicine*, 69, 378–384.

Prainsack, B. & Buyx, A. 2012. Solidarity in contemporary bioethics – Towards a new approach. *Bioethics*, 26, 343–350.

Preciado Serrano, M. D. L., Salas Sanchez, E., Franco Chavez, S. & Vazquez Goni, J. 2010. Psychosocial risk, burnout and emotional labour exhaustion in physicians of a charity institution. *Revista Cubana de Salud y Trabajo*, 11, 3–8.

Raab, K. 2014. Mindfulness, self-compassion, and empathy among health care professionals: A review of the literature. *Journal of Health Care Chaplaincy*, 20, 95–108.

Riess, H., Kelley, J. M., Bailey, R. W., Dunn, E. J. & Phillips, M. 2012. Empathy training for resident physicians: A randomized controlled trial of a neuroscience-informed curriculum. *Journal of General Internal Medicine*, 27, 1280–1286.

Segal, E. A. 2011. Social empathy: A model built on empathy, contextual understanding, and social responsibility that promotes social justice. *Journal of Social Service Research*, 37, 266–277.

Spiro, H. 1992. What is empathy and can it be taught? *Annals of Internal Medicine*, 116, 843–846.

Stjernø, S. 2009. *Solidarity in Europe: The History of an Idea*, Cambridge: Cambridge University Press.

Stürmer, S., Snyder, M. & Omoto, A. M. 2005. Prosocial emotions and helping: The moderating role of group membership. *Journal of Personality and Social Psychology*, 88, 532.

Ter Meulen, R. 2015. Solidarity and justice in health care: A critical analysis of their relationship. *Diametros*, 43, 1–20.

Titmuss, R. M. 1976. *Commitment to Welfare*, London: Allen and Unwin.

Titmuss, R. M. & Seldon, A. 1968. Commitment to welfare*. *Social Policy & Administration*, 2, 196–200.

Tsao, P. & Yu, C. H. 2016. "There's no billing code for empathy" – Animated comics remind medical students of empathy: A qualitative study. *BMC Medical Education*, 16, 204.

Wagner, P., Hendrich, J., Moseley, G. & Hudson, V. 2007. Defining medical professionalism: A qualitative study. *Medical Education*, 41, 288–294.

Wald, H. S. 2015. Professional identity (trans)formation in medical education: Reflection, relationship, resilience. *Academic Medicine*, 90, 701–706.

Wiklund Gustin, L. & Wagner, L. 2013. The butterfly effect of caring – clinical nursing teachers' understanding of self-compassion as a source to compassionate care. *Scandinavian Journal of Caring Sciences*, 27, 175–183.

Zinn, W. 1993. The empathic physician. *Archives of Internal Medicine*, 153, 306–312.

11 Accounting for ethics

Is there a market for morals in healthcare?

Andrew Papanikitas

> Nature, when she formed man for society, endowed him with original desire to please, and an original aversion to offend his brethren. She taught him to feel pleasure in their favourable, and pain in their unfavourable regard. She rendered their approbation most flattering and agreeable to him for its own sake; and their disapprobation most mortifying and offensive.
>
> Adam Smith, *The Theory of Moral Sentiments* (1759)

Introduction

In this chapter, I do two things: I will reflect on previous chapters in this volume as I discuss how any form of market presents ethical issues for healthcare professionals. My inference is that these are best navigated with some form of educational input based on sound scholarship and an intelligent pedagogical approach. I will also discuss possible and ideal forms of a market in healthcare ethics which serves a wider healthcare sector that in turn serves society.

My starting premise is therefore that any kind of healthcare market generates a need for ethical activity, and I expand upon this in the first section of the chapter. I will not attempt to argue that healthcare needs ethics because that argument has already been well-made by others. In so far as healthcare needs ethics, however, I will ask what provision is and ought to be made for that need in a healthcare marketplace.

Just as some form of market exists in healthcare, I will assume that there is a form of market in medical ethics. I will also take the next step in asking what form this market for ethics in healthcare can and ought to take. The form of market that exists for healthcare ethics is influenced by several factors, including the perceived need for healthcare ethics, the visibility of activity in this arena, and the availability of resources for those activities. My argument seeks to marry ideas from moral philosophy, educational theory and the social sciences.

Whilst I discuss the place of ethics research and education in a healthcare market, it is difficult to restrict definitions of either ethics or markets. Many kinds of market operate in a healthcare system. It may of course be worthwhile at times to consider what kind of market operates in specific examples. In the context where

I currently practice, British primary healthcare, for example, Iliffe describes two types of market in operation (Iliffe, 2008).

> The type I [market] is based on a 'needs-led' model of purchasing and is sometimes called an 'industrial' market. In this market the purchaser is a health authority, acting on behalf of a geographically defined, resident population . . . the type II market (sometimes called a 'retail' market) is based on 'demand-led' model. Here, the market existed between providers and those GPs who had chosen to hold their own budget for hospital and community care, the fundholders.
>
> (Iliffe, 2008)

This somewhat simplistic account nonetheless serves as a useful reminder that not all markets are about the satisfaction of individual preferences. Like other aspects of healthcare, 'healthcare ethics' is purchased by third party payers and healthcare professionals on a needs-led basis. It is also purchased directly by healthcare professionals on a retail or 'demand-led' basis.

Ethics also has multiple meanings and forms, including theory, rules and an understanding of right, wrong and how to live well (Dowie and Martin, 2011; Dowie, 2011). Those meanings will alter depending on what one wants from ethics. For example, a policy-maker who desires a dependable workforce that responds in similar ways to similar challenges may be interested in rules. A practitioner who wants to reconcile competing values may be interested in how to balance goods, harms and choices in ways that are fair.

I will ask whether markets themselves distort professional ethics activity by focussing on novel issues in medical research and policy-level work. By contrast, much of the need and indeed demand for ethics education and support arises in everyday healthcare practice.

1. Need and demand as the basis for a market in healthcare ethics

1.1 Work as 'moral weakness'

Professionals of any sort who operate in any healthcare market need something to prevent the goal of acquiring wealth and status from entirely eclipsing other worthy goals, or causing unjust harms to others. Other chapters in this volume make explicit reference to Adam Smith's *Wealth of Nations*. I will not dwell on it, save to note Smith's observation that because people actively pursue the advancement of their material or social position, individuals may act in ways that have hurtful consequences for others (Skinner, 1986). *Wealth of Nations*, and influential business-ethics texts that follow from it, have in the past been narrowly interpreted to suggest that markets are best unregulated, and that unfettered self-interest will result in overall societal good – famously described using Smith's metaphor of an 'invisible hand'. This is of course only a part of Smith's social system. James and Rassekh argue that to properly understand Smith's political economy, one must also have studied his moral philosophy lest his overall social system be misinterpreted. They criticise readings of Smith and Milton Friedman in business texts that interpret 'self-interest' in *Wealth of Nations* narrowly, as unbridled selfishness (James and Rassekh, 2000). For Smith and subsequent authors, self-interest not only encompasses something which can be described as conscience, but it is also limited by notions of fair play and by legislation. The simple but powerful point is that the need for markets to be tempered by morality is well-recognised, including by 'foundational' authors such as Adam Smith.

The tension between economic self-interest and morality in healthcare is nicely illustrated by the example of English general practice. General practices in England have historically been paid by on a fee-for-service or subscription basis, capitation (payment based on patient list-size), incentivised activities and now a mixture of some or all of the above. GPs serve as a good example because the business model for NHS General Practice has, since the foundation of the NHS, been that of a small business subcontracting to provide primary care services. GP Partners are owners of the aforementioned small business and therefore materially affected by the difference between income and expenditure. If patient-centredness really is a core ethical feature of general practice, then GPs who claim to be patient-centred ought to prioritise this above financial incentives. By contrast, without professional ethics (including patient-centredness), any system of payment for GP services might result in maximisation of income in preference to patient welfare. Roland illustrates this in the following table (Roland, 2012).

However, the discussion around payment-for-performance incentives should not be separated from the general discussion of GP's interests as employers, employees and citizens who themselves need to make a living from their vocation. The income that practices receive is expected to provide for staff, the premises and equipment. GP partners do not earn a fixed salary but have to pay themselves out of the surplus. Toon notes the dissonance between the plethora of literature on making a success of general practice as a business and the literature emerging from

Table 11.1 How any payment structure can be misused in the absence of professional ethics?

Payment method		What doctors would do if they did not behave in line with their professional principles
Salary	Pay independent of workload or quality	As little as possible for as few people as possible
Capitation	Pay according to the number of people on a doctor's list	As little as possible for as many people as possible
Fee-for-service	Pay for individual items of care	As much as possible, whether or not it helped the patient
Pay for performance	Pay for meeting quality targets	A limited range of commendable tasks, but nothing else

journals and the Royal College of General Practitioners (Toon, 1994). He points out that academic scholarship predominantly treats doctors as platonic gentlemen of independent means, whose sole concern is to decide morally and empirically how best to occupy their time. Clearly this view is a caricature, but it illustrates the need for a bridge between abstract ideals and reality. The ethic of patient-centredness is a core feature of GP training – but preparation for how this ethic will be tested in practice seems far less core. Ethics must serve patients but must also acknowledge the interests of GPs as employees and owners of small businesses.

Previous chapters in this volume have already signalled that healthcare generates moral demands upon those who work in the sector. The word 'Work' is significant here, as distinct from 'Play.' The range of monetised activities and types of healthcare market capture the value of work and allow that work to be materially rewarded. For most professionals involved in healthcare around the world, these are occupations on which their livelihoods depend. This dependency itself presents a source of moral weakness. I recently saw a satirical cartoon of a politician visiting a hospital.* "Where's the money?" he asks – the implication being that he sees it as a money-making enterprise rather than an institution in service of the sick. The discomfiting answer is, "everywhere." As pointed out in this volume, work is transvalued into economic terms (money) in various ways. Feiler and Herring present ways of monetising (respectively) instances of treatable illness with matched treatments (Feiler, 2018) and episodes of care (Herring, 2018). The danger with both is that the person receiving healthcare or care more broadly risks becoming 'merely' a means to access a defined financial amount and less an 'end.' The itemisation of activities for economic purposes risks end-users of healthcare being 'short changed,' but it also risks toxic (sometimes literally) over-testing and overtreatment. The latter case is made by Jani and myself (Jani and Papanikitas, 2018) in our discussion of defensive medicine. Overly or badly-marketised healthcare, we argue, creates a social pressure on doctors and others to practice in ways that reduce risk and uncertainty for healthcare providers, whilst compromising the quality of care for patients. Some writers go so far as to say that any connection between financial interests and decision-making represents a conflict of interest (Epstein, 2014), and that any method of incentivising practice can be subverted in ways that undermine their purpose (Roland, 2012). If these and other accounts tell us anything, it is that no current manner of remunerating healthcare work is perfect (yet).

The economisation of healthcare, implicit in the economisation of illness, treatment, care and patient populations that is illustrated in the preceding chapters, is just one aspect of healthcare that renders people vulnerable to unethical practice. Patient safety and healthcare quality are however ostensible reasons why healthcare ethics is researched, encoded in policy and mission-statements, taught and learned. The presence of perceived necessity drives a market for concepts, codes and education.

One answer to the problem of healthcare providers' interests is championed in this volume by Epstein: do away with markets entirely in favour of a society that takes from each according to their ability and gives to each according to their need (Epstein, 2018). The problem with this solution is twofold: first, it would not necessarily account for moral challenges that are unrelated to economic welfare of the healthcare professional; second, the solution does not help those who do not live (or have no prospect of living) in such a utopia – practical healthcare ethics being not so much a source of answers to the question, "What should we do?" but a robust set of approaches to the question, "What should we do *now*?" The contrast between these two questions lies in the word 'now.' To decry the moral failures that have given rise to an ethical issue is of little help in solving the issue which has arisen.

1.2 Ethical antidotes to healthcare markets – the basis for a market in ethics?

In *The Theory of Moral Sentiments*, Adam Smith argued that individuals in society are subject to two jurisdictions that control their feelings and actions; the jurisdiction of the external spectator and the jurisdiction of their own consciences. In discussing the right ways to live with variously marketised healthcare, some authors in this volume espouse internal qualities (or virtues) for healthcare professionals. Others discuss ways in which professionals may engage with (using Adam Smith's vernacular) kinds of 'external spectator', whether entering into covenants or coming under the scrutiny of an ethics committee. Perhaps this echoes Smith's distinct discussions of actions that follow one's conscience and actions that might be deemed praiseworthy. In *What Money Can't Buy*, Sandel cites Arrow in highlighting arguments that ethics (in a manner that resembles virtue or conscience) should factor in only as a scarce resource, and that pricing mechanisms should be used where possible so that the well of human goodness does not run dry (Sandel, 2012; Arrow, 1972). I propose that activity which aims at the moral strengthening of individuals and institutions, especially that which is illustrated by authors in this volume, cannot reliably and sustainably exist unless it is supported by intellectual and material resources. In the provision of those resources lies a market.

Walsh, Misselbrook and Kerasidou and Horn (2018) are implicit and explicit that a moral education will enable healthcare professionals to resist the anti-social, destructively selfish elements of the market environment. For example, ethics education has a potential role in the prevention of financial incentives becoming ends in themselves (Kerasidou and Horn, 2018; Misselbrook, 2018; Walsh, 2018). They argue that healthcare professionals may and should exercise human virtues in order to flourish in whatever form of market they offer their services. Kerasidou and Horn argue that empathy is not only possible in marketised healthcare, but also essential for good practice, with benefits not only for individual patients, but the emotional wellbeing of clinicians themselves (Kerasidou and Horn, 2018). Empathy, however, is difficult to measure and impossible to count in a manner that can be itemised for billing. Misselbrook is more expansive, arguing that clinicians need to develop virtues, and that a virtuous clinician moderates acts of beneficence with survival in the workplace, not least by earning enough to support themselves and, where relevant, colleagues as well (Misselbrook, 2018). Virtues aim at flourishing in practice and the flourishing is both in perfecting one's art and succeeding at one's business. This means striving to practise with excellence and acting rightly according to reason – something that is not necessarily easy. Empathy and virtues appear as internal qualities, personal values that might drive an individual to practice in a way that is morally right from the perspective of one's own conscience.

Others in this volume expand on ways in which healthcare professionals might seek different kinds of approval. Frith discusses organisational ethics, manifest as policy and as people with expertise and a mandate to hold organisation and its employees true to its espoused values (Frith, 2018). Hordern discusses the potential role of a covenant between those who offer healthcare, those who receive care and wider society (Hordern, 2018).

I invite the reader to consider the idea that the antidotes to moral weakness that authors in this volume offer such as codes, covenants, collegiality and conscience (and useful concepts in general) are all products in a market place of sorts. Healthcare ethics is 'sold' as being of benefit to populations, institutions and to individuals (patients and healthcare professionals). For populations, healthcare ethics promises to promote the quality of healthcare and patient safety. Those in charge of medical school curricula and specialist training programmes make some (but not much) time and resource available for ethics. For institutions, healthcare ethics promises to promote the kind of workforce that will generate a good reputation, work hard and diligently, and refuse to obey commands that are misguided or wrong in a moral sense. This manifests as mission-statements, codes of practice, guidelines and, far less often than in the academic education setting, education and training. Individual patients arguably benefit from interaction with healthcare professionals who respect their personhood and aim to encourage their flourishing. Individual healthcare professionals flourish in their jobs when the job aligns with their values (Toon, 2009; Papanikitas, 2017b)

If healthcare ethics, construed broadly, offers such benefits, then who is expected to pay for these activities? Plausible candidates include: the taxpayer, institutions, charitable bodies and healthcare professionals themselves. Patients or 'end-users' might plausibly contribute in that some notional part of their fee might go towards ethics education in the same way that it might go towards medical indemnity or mandatory training of some sort. This means that healthcare ethics activity is largely commissioned by institutions. Where there is a perceived need for knowledge and skill that are in some way essential to practice, or that benefit a population, a purchaser might obtain research and education in order to allow this to happen. For example, purchasing authority A purchases education for practitioner B in order to benefit patient C. Or it may be sought after by healthcare professionals themselves.

An example of healthcare ethics 'commissioned' lies in the ethical frameworks adopted by the clinical commissioning groups (CCGs) of England. Commissioning by institutions tends towards an industrial market or needs-led approach and therefore favours tangible products with tangible benefits, preferably at scale – a 'process' applicable to all CCGs therefore represents a product to be commissioned. Ethical frameworks for commissioning are statements combining law and societal values and are in essence just such processes to which CCGs might refer. One such document has been produced by the Priorities Support Unit, an NHS organisation that has since become an NHS consultancy organisation called 'Solutions for public health' (NHS, 2017b; NHS, 2017a). Another, more complex, document is offered by the Royal College of General Practitioners (Oswald and Cox, 2011). The need for documents is straightforward – a CCG is accountable in particular ways and has certain duties. A document outlining these duties and accountabilities is therefore an easy solution. A problem with such pieces of work is that there is no guarantee that commissioners will be aware of or read either document. However, this chapter is not focussing on policy and rules but responding to several chapters in this volume suggesting that something more fundamental is needed than rules.

Interestingly both the ethical framework for commissioning and the RCGP ethical guidance for commissioners offer principles rather than rules. As previous authors in this volume have intimated – healthcare professionals need the space and support to develop wisdom, to maintain empathy and compassion, and to have the courage to practice patient-centred medicine amid the perverse pressures of the market. The solution, I propose, lies in education. Healthcare commissioning has been described as a four stage process (Cox and Papanikitas, 2017).

- Identify the need (referred to as needs assessment)
- Identify capacity to meet the need (referred to as tendering)
- Delivery of service from that capacity (referred to as procurement)
- Evaluation of the service (referred to as contract management). Evaluation should be linked to ways of improving or replacing a service which is inadequate.

Can a need for healthcare ethics education be captured in a way that a CCG would recognise? The avoidance of litigation, the promise of better decisions that are more publicly defensible, the value in professionals who are less distressed by the decisions they make, might well be captured as needs worth addressing. How does one tender to meet those needs? Some resource allocation panels buy the time (or solicit the voluntary service) of an ethicist. Another approach might be to arrange training for CCG members, either 'in house' or by subsidising attendance on a course. Evaluation of such a service is a harder proposition. How does one find evidence that education improves healthcare worker resilience, improves ethico-legal defensibility of decisions or increases good in the system? Ironically CCG commissioners may conscientiously forego ethics education on the basis that it does not have a sufficient scientific evidence base and cannot (yet) be linked to measurable outcomes. Ethics activities risk being perceived in the same way as complementary and alternative therapies – with its users claiming benefit in ways that are hard to tangibly measure (Papanikitas, 2017a). If they cannot be framed as 'needs' then they may be provided on a 'demand' basis. For example, commissioners who see the relevance of such an activity might enrol themselves in a course on ethics or philosophy applied to healthcare.

2. The form of the market in healthcare ethics

In the previous section I mentioned some potential needs and demands that might offer a 'market' for healthcare ethics. I now consider the form of that market in terms of the products on offer – or the 'capacity to meet the need' alluded to in the simplified commissioning stages.

> Money is the stuff of life; it is the medium of exchange that we use to buy food, clothes, warmth in the winter, cool in the summer, and the fuel that moves us around the planet. Of course money makes the world go 'round, but does it . . . make bioethics go 'round?
>
> (De Vries and Keirns, 2008)

If money makes bioethics go around then the same must hold true for healthcare ethics, whether these activities entail research into the dilemmas of practice, education for healthcare professionals, providing decision-making support to clinicians or writing policy documents. In so far as these activities are either paid or cost money (someone gets paid for something), there arguably exists a market for ethics in healthcare.

Healthcare ethics is sold in two key ways: it is sold as theoretical content (or intellectual product) or as more tangible products. These more tangible products are economised in three basic ways: as documentation (such as books and papers), as tasks (such as research projects and classes) or as time spent (such as an hourly or other sessional rate paid to an advisor or tutor). This is a gross oversimplification because the economic costs of a market in healthcare also lie for example in the value of time spent learning as well as the teacher's fee. I am going to concentrate on two markets as they relate to healthcare, albeit briefly, here – a market in knowledge and its application, and, separately, a market in ethics education. Space and time do not permit a consideration of healthcare ethics consultancy, of ethics consultation and review in the clinical setting or of other manifestations of a market in healthcare ethics.

2.1 From knowledge to policy – translational ethics as we know it

Much of the paid activity in healthcare ethics is in academic contexts – going under the heading of 'Bioethics.' Research projects which may be theoretical or empirical or a combination are usually paid for by an interested third party such as a funding body, charity, government institution or even business (De Vries and Keirns, 2008). Some funding bodies aim to support new, innovative or otherwise compelling ideas – such as the Wellcome Trust (WT, 2017). Other funding bodies may support research that meets with a particular ideology or agenda – for examples disease-specific charities. Much of the funding activity in bioethics concentrates on new developments in health sciences, as suggested by Butcher in a Wellcome Trust blog post (Butcher, 2011).

> A lot of attention in biomedical ethics focuses – rightly – on experimental and exciting new developments in biomedical science such as human

enhancement, genetics and neuroscience to name a few. But while these topics are of vital importance, they often have little relevance to healthcare professionals' everyday working lives.

(Butcher, 2011)

Relevance or utility are key elements in any academic field's argument for material resources. This is illustrated in the argument that a medical context has 'saved' the life of ethics and has given back a seriousness and human relevance to the subject of ethics (Toulmin, 1982). The same argument is repeated a decade later in the context of the conjunction between ethics and social sciences (Hoffmaster, 1992). By contrast, with the idea that ethics might be seen as a somewhat dry and unexciting subject that might not attract large amounts of funding or public attention, Toulmin describes the increasing prestige of bioethics in America:

Before long moral philosophers (or as they barbarously began to be called, 'ethicists') found that they were as liable as the economists to be called on to write 'op ed' pieces for the New York Times, or to testify before congressional committees.

(Toulmin, 1982)

According to Toulmin, the new medical ethics saved the life of ethics as an overlooked and under-resourced discipline by applying ethics outside the classroom. Toulmin argues that ethicists applied rationality to – and therefore resolved arguments over – matters of public policy, i.e. they made themselves useful and placed themselves in public view. They achieved this by colonising an area of public interest: medical ethics. Policy relevance and policy influence are certainly reasons to claim funding in applications to the major charitable institutions. Both Toulmin and Hoffmaster above refer to a saving of the academic endeavour in intellectual terms, but there is undeniably a saving in a material sense also.

In her Wellcome Blog on 'Unsexy ethics,' Butcher highlights two studies that might contrast with experimental and exciting new developments in bioethics: one study focusses on researchers' constructions of ethics in the context of embryonic stem cell biology, and the other on leadership and organisational ethics. Whilst both studies have produced innovative and compelling ideas with clear policy relevance, they serve to illustrate a point – they are not 'unsexy'. Policy relevance and policy influence (impact) are key selling-points for academic studies in healthcare ethics. Both grants which to Butcher refers represent costs of research and livelihood for researchers. In order to survive in the 'business' of research, researchers must find people who are prepared to pay for their activities, or they must pursue activities that people are prepared to pay for. Dunn et al. highlight this in their discussion of themes arising at a conference for PhD students and early career researchers in Bioethics:

we need to be able to define ourselves in ways that allow us to identify with, and be able to apply successfully for, specific funding streams and jobs . . . If we are going to obtain funding for our research, we need to know that funding bodies will take our applications seriously.

(Dunn et al., 2008)

Policy-relevance is a natural kind of 'impact' or 'purchased outcome' for ethics because ethics can exist as both a form of scholarship and as a form of regulation. As such, it can be both something that people learn about and a boundary to what professions can and ought to do. Policy is critically important, I have already argued, but not enough by itself to sustain good practice in a healthcare market-place. Policies, rules, guidelines and codes of practice refer to values in ways that sometimes fail to account for their meanings and allude implicitly to values in ways that fail to allow for their critical analysis. This has been illustrated by a number of writers. In discussing translational ethics, Cribb suggests that ethics enacted are re-shaped from their original design by a number of social factors including political and local agendas (Cribb, 2010). Fulford and colleagues critique what they call quasi-legal ethics, the tendency towards an ever-fatter rule book and draconian guidelines that are more honoured in the breach than the observance (Fulford et al., 2002). Heath and others comment on the 'Reality gap', a tendency of those in charge to inflate duties without considering how they might be achieved (Heath, 2008). In this volume, Misselbrook illustrates this in relation to the Francis Report on the poor care delivered in Mid-Staffordshire. The report suggested that staff were unable to provide compassionate care because of the pressures of work and sheer number of guidelines, and then went on to propose additional guidelines. A healthcare ethics market that concentrates predominantly on the generation of new knowledge but neglects education offers only a partial good.

Research can offer insight into the development of ethics in the historical health-care market place. Research into manners, etiquette and rules of good conduct for healthcare professionals can offer such insights. In this volume, Misselbrook also makes reference to several accounts of medical power over patients – such as Friedson's account of 'ethicality'. Friedson argued that by making claims of service orientation – serving the sick – doctors were able to avoid regulation and maintain status and professional autonomy. Frith (in citing Wilson's account) also suggests that the development of medical ethics allowed the medical profession to retain status and power (Wilson, 2014a, 2014b; Frith, 2018). These conform to a narrative of espoused ethics being good for business but also to a narrative of healthcare ethics that is above all about the power of doctors.

Research can usefully challenge this common narrative of ethics and raise questions of current relevance – McCullough, for example, critiques accounts of Hippocratic ethics as paternalist by suggesting that duties promoted in the Hippocratic corpus are about protecting trade secrets and not giving away one's livelihood:

the text . . . in which the physician is exhorted to prepare his remedies in secret and not tell the sick individual what is in them, has nothing to do with paternalism. It has everything to do with protecting trade secrets and one's market-share. Ingredients used by ancient physicians were not regulated by a

Food and Drug Administration and could be found in households or markets. If the sick individual or house-hold member observed the physician preparing an ointment or elixir, then the sick individual could dismiss the physician from service and instruct his servants to make the ointment or elixir. The passage quoted . . . is about prudence, the virtue that instructs the physician to identify his legitimate self-interests (preserving trade secrets that are essential to continued employment) and act to protect them.

(McCullough, 2011)

Such research is of limited value to healthcare, however, unless it influences policy and practice, perhaps by informing more realistic policy or fostering reflexivity in healthcare professionals through education. Relevance in the 'real world' outside the classroom is one way in which academic fields and disciplines are justified.

2.2 *Education*

If there is a market for ethics education in healthcare, then it is worth considering who the customer is. There are two ways of thinking about customers – those who purchase services and those who use services. To begin, I consider the public, healthcare employers and healthcare professionals themselves.

Ethics education for healthcare professionals is not something generally purchased by patients or directly by the public. They may take an educational (e.g. a public philosophy course) or informational (following the news) or more voyeuristic interest (tragic dilemmas make good stories). They may have direct interest, by virtue of a professional activity (being on a clinical ethics committee or a patient participation and involvement in research representative) or having a stake in a given case. They do not represent a group to whom medical ethics teachers currently sell their time and expertise. Yet the public, broadly speaking, do stand to gain from conscientious professionals who pursue goals beyond the narrow accumulation of personal wealth, power and prestige. Governments via the devolved agencies that coordinate educational activities might act on the public's behalf and encourage, or at least not discourage, the resourcing of some teaching for healthcare professionals, such as the aforementioned GPs. Charities acting on behalf of patients might also be minded to fund such activities for similar reasons.

Employers represent a more significant market. What employer would not want the kind of workforce that will generate a good reputation, work hard and diligently and refuse to obey commands that are misguided or harmful to patients and the employer's reputation? They might, however be reluctant to commission time spent on activities that will not be linked to a measurable increase in revenue. A surgical skill by contrast can be 'put to work' and billed for. In addition, they may not wish to encourage independent thinking or even conscientious objection from their employees. There is also an implication that, alongside other connections to the humanities, healthcare ethics is a leisure activity. Thinking time is seen as unproductive time – time at work must be spent doing; thinking can be done at home.

Finally, healthcare professionals themselves may have an interest in purchasing ethics education. Many of the benefits of ethics education are general welfare benefits – a recent pilot study of graduates from an intercalated course in medical ethics and law found that students gained general transferable skills such as presentation and self-directed learning but also 'character' benefits such as confidence (Ives et al., 2013). The same study interestingly also discussed costs to the learner, such as delaying one's earnings by a year as a result of doing the course. Elsewhere I have argued that healthcare professionals learn about ethics for a number of reasons: it may be a necessary component of accreditation as a practitioner, it could serve to provide specific skills for roles in leadership, teaching, research, management and commissioning, and may offer survival skills for practice – whether in making better and more confident decisions or understanding how much moral agency one has and engaging with ethical issues (Papanikitas and Spicer, 2017). It is hard to assign a value to such activities other than what they cost to provide and what people are willing or able to pay for them.

Education provision, accordingly, may be broadly orientated towards different purposes and, therefore, towards different kinds of purchasers. Eisner argued that there are five basic orientations to a curriculum. He refers to cognitive processes, academic rationalism, personal relevance, social adaptation and social reconstruction and curriculum as technology (Eisner, 1985). All these orientations have a bearing on ethics education and point to different kinds of markets.

- An orientation towards the development of cognitive processes emphasises the belief that curriculum and teaching strategy should foster the student's ability to think and reason.
- Academic rationalism argues that the function of education is to foster the intellectual growth of students in those subject matters most worthy of study.
- Personal relevance emphasises the primacy of personal meaning for the learner and the educator's responsibility to make such meaning possible.
- Social adaptation and social reconstruction collectively are an orientation that derives its aims and content from an analysis of the society that education is designed to serve. Social adaptation aimed to prepare learners to meet society's ostensible needs. Social reconstruction aims at learners who will recognise and improve upon the deficiencies in society.
- Curriculum as technology is an orientation that conceives of curriculum planning as a technical undertaking, relating means to ends that have already been formulated.

I suggest to the reader that orientation toward cognitive processes, academic rationalism and personal relevance largely favour a retail market, and that social adaptation/reconstruction and curriculum as technology largely favour the institutional/industrial purchaser. This, in effect, represents a divide between 'education as personal flourishing' and 'education to shape the learner for a function in society'.

I offer, as a case study, ethics education in the professional journey of a UK General Practitioner – based partly on my own academic doctoral thesis in medical education. As one can clearly see, the purchaser of the education is not necessarily the same as the recipient. Many of the activities are commissioned to adapt the student and then doctor for medicine and then general practice.

- Undergraduate ethics education is present in all UK medical schools but varies in its delivery and assessment. There is a consensus statement on ethics and law in lieu of a national curriculum (Stirrat et al., 2010). However, recent research shows that this curriculum is variably and sometimes poorly implemented (Brooks and Bell, 2016) and some question whether ethics education at medical school is useful (Sokol, 2016).
- The Foundation Years curriculum has a section on ethics and law. It focusses on specific practical issues rather than fundamental ethics and values. Foundation year doctors may have one session of formal ethics education of variable relevance (Sokol, 2010; Parker, 2017).
- Membership of the Royal College of General Practitioners RCGP: There was a curriculum statement on ethics and values until 2012. Ethics and values are now threaded into the various parts of the curriculum. Issues appear on various statements, particularly the core statement on being a GP. Understanding and application of ethics can be assessed explicitly in work-place based assessments though it is not an absolute requirement for accreditation. It is also tested with other aspects of professionalism in the clinical skills assessment. However, there is no standard on teaching ethics for teachers or formal criteria for teaching of ethics in General Practice training. This occurs, when it does, in discussion between trainees and trainers, in one or at most two teaching sessions on a 'half day release' (Gillies, 2009).
- Unofficial education includes: What GPs bring from their societal background and upbringing including from religion and school. The hidden curriculum from medical school and junior doctor can be influential. Role-modelling – good and bad – may also influence attitudes and values. This hidden curriculum is sometimes tackled by offering education to those who act as role models.
- Educational offerings for qualified GPs include an assortment of higher degrees, postgraduate courses, certificates and diplomas. These are aimed at supporting various roles of GPs such as teaching, leadership, and clinical commissioning, but also survival skills for daily practice (Papanikitas and Spicer, 2017).

In the above case, the need to ensure accreditation presents both an industrial market (ethics is included in the training programme) and a retail market (students, trainees and practitioners seek out courses). The above case also illustrates the potential for needs not to be met if there is insufficient demand to run a course or insufficient visibility in the curriculum to include ethics in a training programme.

In contrast to academic research in healthcare ethics, which is largely conducted by professional academics, ethics education seems more of a 'cottage industry'; much of the teaching happening on a semi-voluntary basis. Whilst I have portrayed education as a poor cousin to research, I am aware that there is a lack of data to support what ostensibly is an empirical claim. It is interesting to note that data are available on who buys bioethics research, though even this is incomplete and largely focusses on empirical research (involving the gathering of data) (De Vries and Keirns, 2008). De Vries and Keirns' special issue of the *American Journal of Bioethics* – "Who buys bioethics?" – makes for sober and inconclusive reading. Data are needed, however, on the value (both in societal and economic terms) of activities in bioethics and, for our purposes, healthcare ethics. Data are also needed on the quality of the market – what activities come under a banner of healthcare ethics, who pays for them and why do they pay for them? Are there any risks or harms we should be wary of that are analogous to other 'harmful' aspects of a healthcare market?

3. The dark side of a market in healthcare ethics

There are a number of critiques of bioethics, and some of them are relevant to a discussion of markets and ethics in healthcare: Ethics is a way in which the strong (socially speaking) oppress the weak (Hoeyer, 2006); ethics can be ideological or corrupt (Epstein, 2008) and ethics craves sensationalism and novelty because that is where the funding is (Papanikitas et al., 2011).

3.1 Ethics as a means of oppression

The idea of bioethics as a potential abuse of power is one that is touched upon in this volume by Epstein (Epstein, 2018). In this account, the bioethics may be oppressive in the following ways: Ethics and morality are about service orientation in any given workforce and therefore can be used in ways that are exploitative by employers. If the need for healthcare far exceeds its current capacity to provide services in any given instance then doctors and other staff will routinely give more than they are contracted for. The recent UK Junior doctors' strike is a case in point, as the only legitimate public argument for a strike for a group of paid professionals appeared to be the argument that working conditions were unsafe for patients (Toynbee et al., 2016). That the new conditions were unsafe *for doctors* or unjust in any other way was generally considered secondary. Furthermore, many essential services continued to run during the strike as senior doctors did the work of the junior doctors. Early on in the strikes, a 'work to rule,' where junior doctors worked their contracted duties and no more, was considered to be a form of strike, in and of itself.

The other way in which bioethics can be seen as an exercise of power is in the making of rules and guidelines. I have previously alluded to the concept of boundary-work (Gieryn, 1999; Gieryn, 1983). Ethical boundary-work is where a group of professionals define what is ethical in ways that permit some people (arguably those who are already established in positions of power) to continue practising and to deny 'the market' to those who are unable to meet the same standards (Wainwright et al., 2006). Whilst medical research ethics ostensibly protects research participants, it also serves as a barrier for new and less supported researchers.

3.2 Ethics as cultural imperialism

Epstein suggests that we should be just as concerned by bioethics in the service of ideology as bioethics as a legalistic means of achieving a convenient end, or coming up with good excuses for less praiseworthy agendas. He provocatively titles his paper, "Tell us what you want to do and we'll tell you how to do it ethically." The healthcare ethics marketplace offers many ways to flourish and seek righteousness – there is fierce debate about which is the best or the right one. There are a number of ethical approaches that pervade healthcare in the United Kingdom: deontology, utilitarianism and consequentialism virtues, values-based approaches, libertarian philosophies, rights-based approaches and ethical contractarianism, feminist approaches and others. Some of these may be promoted because a grant awarding body or institution wishes to promote healthcare ethics in line with their ethos or political orientation. Some approaches to healthcare ethics may have achieved a status as a 'brand plus method' such as Values-based practice (Petrova et al., 2006) or the four principles of Anglo-American bioethics (Gillon, 2003). Whilst that status per se is not bad, the superficial adoption and poor use of those methods is something to be guarded against. Moreover, a 'brand' may eclipse other approaches even when they are manifestly appropriate. The concern about cultural imperialism arises when an approach is used because it is favoured by a powerful cultural group – the four principles being used (for example) because they come from America, or Values Based Practice being favoured because it has been adopted by the RCGP.

3.3 Ethics that craves novelty and only follows the money

Finally, bioethics research has perennially focussed on that which is perceived as new in healthcare. Funding for bioethics research can often arise as part of, or connected to, funding for biomedical research – translational research in the biosciences is looked upon more favourably when there is a serious attempt to grapple with the ethical legal and social aspects (or issues – the common acronym is ELSI or ELSA) of the new thing being developed. The collateral danger is that where there is no large translational research project there is little funding, and therefore academic interest in work on the ethics of practice. Similarly, the empirical 'turn' in bioethics coincides with work that can be itemised and therefore (arguably) more easily monetised. In many ways thinking, writing and even teaching no longer count as work, but instead they are worthy voluntary activities peripheral to research and healthcare practice.

Healthcare ethics is embodied in people and part of a market in healthcare, offering activities such as research, education and advice on policy and practice. I have already argued that those who embody healthcare ethics are not untouched by market forces.

4. Conclusion

In this chapter, I have used markets as a tool with which to start a conversation about how healthcare ethics manifests as an aspect of healthcare. This picks up on a theme that runs thought this book – that markets can be used as a way to understand both the materiality of healthcare and the way that morality is applied to and in healthcare.

An exchange of goods (a market) takes place in any healthcare system. Any form of market presents ethical issues for healthcare professionals – these are issues that are both related (issues of markets) and unrelated (issues in markets) to the economic drivers of healthcare. I have suggested that these are best navigated with sound policy and good education. Healthcare environments that meaningfully support ethical practice need to be understood and supported. As markets are framed around needs, these needs imply a market in healthcare ethics. Such a market needs theory and data; it also needs activity to put new and existing theory and data to good use. At the outset, I suggested that ethics research and education in particular are intrinsic to a healthcare market – ethics education and research is itself purchased and conducted within that market. Other activities such as consultancy and clinical or research ethics review in the healthcare setting are also intrinsic and merit further study. That healthcare ethics is for sale is not in doubt – and the potential abuse (whether through deliberate choice or ignorance) of healthcare ethics is a worrying phenomenon that must be taken seriously.

This chapter has not tackled the question of whether ethics in healthcare ought to be commodified in the ways I have outlined: documentation, tasks and time. Should ethics research and education, consultancy etc. be voluntary or leisure activities? This is an area that requires realistic debate – would this threaten standards of provision, and would it, for example, mean that in times of workload pressure crisis everyone was so busy 'doing' that there would be no one to 'think?'

It is also impossible to argue that academic and practical healthcare ethics in its myriad professional forms are entirely untouched by economic considerations. Whether or not ethics ought to be commodified, unless it is appropriately resourced, pressures to concentrate on paid activities in a healthcare market will mean that healthcare ethics research is shaped by whoever is prepared to pay for it. This risks concentration of activity at the frontier, as 'ethicists' participate in a gold rush for funding. It also risks 'Boom and bust' activity where resources are developed in response to a crisis but fail to be sustainable or self-sustaining. A market in healthcare ethics – if it is to effectively serve a broader healthcare market, and ultimately society, must sustain 'everyday' aspects of good healthcare. If it concentrates primarily on policy or on novel technologies it will only offer a partial good, and healthcare ethics education will continue to be haphazardly provided.

For a market in healthcare ethics to work, purchasers must recognise value in healthcare ethics activities, being both the self-interested value of return on investment and the social value of putting good into the world. Providers must offer products that are meaningful to purchasers – and educating the buyer to the necessity of what one offers has a long history in the commercial world – it is called marketing! Work is needed to establish the answer to what has become a 'Holy Grail' of healthcare ethics – "What good does healthcare ethics do?" But questions of who assigns value and how financial value is assigned to such activities need to be addressed because we live in a society where money is the means by which we exchange work for material goods.

4.1 Acknowledgements and a declaration of interest

This chapter has arisen from a number of meetings and conversations convened under the auspices of the Oxford University Healthcare Values Partnership funded by the British Academy and supported by the Nuffield Department of Primary Care Health Sciences. The funding for my post comes from the National Institute of Health Research. Key meetings that contributed to this chapter included a series of research seminars on Markets and Meaning in Healthcare at Harris Manchester College and The Oxford Research Centre for the Humanities as well as a conference at the Royal Society of Medicine (RSM) – "Engaging healthcare: the ethics of markets and a marketplace for ethics?" – held jointly between the Healthcare Values Partnership, The Open Section, and the General Practice and Primary healthcare section. Video recordings of key participant comments and some presentations are available to access on the Healthcare Values Partnership website. I am grateful to Peter Toon and Kim Stillman for initial discussions in development of my ideas on the concept of the healthcare ethics market. I am particularly grateful to Dr Emma McKenzie-Edwards, Professor Joshua Hordern and Dr Therese Feiler for assistance in developing this chapter, and the many others who read or listened and offered feedback.

I am a clinician, but I also have a vested interest in healthcare ethics. I am and have been for a number of years paid to teach, study and write about healthcare ethics. I believe that learning about ethics offers healthcare professionals insight and sometimes agency with respect to ethical issues, and this promises better decision-making and more emotionally resilient professionals.

Note

* With thanks to Miran Epstein for pointing out the cartoon at our writers' meeting.

References

Arrow, K. J. 1972. Gifts and exchanges. *Philosophy and Public Affairs*, 1, 343–362.

Brooks, L. & Bell, D. 2017. Teaching, learning and assessment of medical ethics at the UK medical schools. *Journal of Medical Ethics*, 43, 606–612.

Butcher, F. 2011. *The Appeal of 'Unsexy' Ethics* [Online]. Wordpress. Available: https://blog.wellcome.ac.uk/2011/09/02/the-appeal-of-%e2%80%98unsexy%e2%80%99-ethics/ [Accessed 14/08/17].

Cox, D. & Papanikitas, A. 2017. Difficult decisions: The ethics of GP commissioning. *InnovAiT*, 10, 458–464.

Cribb, A. 2010. Translational ethics? The theory-practice gap in medical ethics. *Journal of Medical Ethics*, 36, 207–210.

De Vries, R. G. & Keirns, C. C. 2008. Does money make bioethics go 'round'? *American Journal of Bioethics*, 8, 65–67.

Dowie, A. & Martin, A. 2011. Clarifying ethics and law in the curriculum. *In:* Gibb, T. (ed.) *Ethics and Law in the Medical Curriculum*. Dundee: Association for Medical Education in Europe.

Dowie, A. L. 2011. Making sense of ethics and law in the medical curriculum. *Medical Teacher*, 33, 384–387.

Dunn, M. C., Gurtin-Broadbent, Z., Wheeler, J. & Ives, J. 2008. Jack of all trades, master of none? Challenges facing junior academic researchers in bioethics. *Clinical Ethics*, 3, 160–163.

Eisner, E. W. 1985. Five basic orientations to the curriculum. *In: The Educational Imagination: On the Design and Evaluation of the School Programs*. New York: Macmillan Publishing.

Epstein, M. 2008. 'Tell us what you want to do, and we'll tell you how to do it ethically' – academic bioethics: Routinely ideological and occasionally corrupt. *American Journal of Bioethics*, 8, 63–65.

Epstein, M. 2014. Disclosure of financial conflicts of interest: cui bono, cui malo? *Journal of the Royal Society of Medicine*, 107, 303.

Epstein, M. 2018. The corruption of medical morality under advanced capitalism. *In:* Feiler, T., Hordern, J. & Papanikitas, A. (eds.) *Marketisation, Ethics and Healthcare: Policy, Practice and Moral Formation*. Abingdon: Routledge.

Feiler, T. 2018. Encoding truths? Diagnosis-related groups and the fragility of the marketisation discourse. *In:* Feiler, T., Hordern, J. & Papanikitas, A. (eds.) *Marketisation, Ethics and Healthcare: Policy, Practice and Moral Formation*. Abingdon: Routledge.

Frith, L. 2018. Organisational ethics: A solution to the challenges of markets in healthcare? *In:* Feiler, T., Hordern, J. & Papanikitas, A. (eds.) *Marketisation, Ethics and Healthcare: Policy, Practice and Moral Formation*. Abingdon: Routledge.

Fulford, K. W. M., Dickenson, D. L. & Murray, T. H. 2002. Many voices: Human values in healthcare ethics. *In:* Fulford, K. W. M., Dickenson, D. L. & Murray, T. H. (eds.) *Healthcare Ethics and Human Values: An Introductory Text with Readings and Case Studies*. Oxford: Blackwell Publishers.

Gieryn, T. F. 1983. Boundary-work and the demarcation of science from non-science: Strains and interests in professional ideologies of scientists. *American Sociological Review*, 48, 781–795.

Gieryn, T. F. 1999. *Cultural Boundaries of Science: Credibility on the Line*, Chicago: University of Chicago Press.

Gillies, J. 2009. Ethics in primary care: Theory and practice. *InnovAIT*, 2, 183–190.

Gillon, R. 2003. Ethics needs principles – four can encompass the rest – and respect for autonomy should be "first among equals". *Journal of Medical Ethics*, 29, 307–312.

Heath, I. 2008. The mystery of general practice. *In: Matters of Life and Death: Key Writings*, Oxford: Radcliffe Publishing.

Herring, J. 2018. Personal budgets: Holding onto the purse strings for fear of something worse. *In:* Feiler, T., Hordern, J. & Papanikitas, A. (eds.) *Marketisation, Ethics and Healthcare: Policy, Practice and Moral Formation*. Abingdon: Routledge.

Hoeyer, K. 2006. "Ethics wars": Reflections on the antagonism between bioethicists and social science observers of biomedicine. *Human Studies*, 29, 203–227.

Hoffmaster, B. 1992. Can ethnography save the life of medical ethics? *Social Science and Medicine*, 35, 1421–1431.

Hordern, J. 2018. Covenant, compassion and marketisation in healthcare: The mastery of Mammon and the service of grace. *In:* Feiler, T., Papanikitas, A. & Hordern, J. (eds.) *Marketisation, Ethics and Healthcare: Policy, Practice and Moral Formation*. Abingdon: Routledge.

Iliffe, S. 2008. The political economy of family medicine. *In: From General Practice to Primary Care: The Industrialisation of Family Medicine*. Oxford: Oxford University Press.

Ives, J., Owens, J. & Cribb, A. 2013. IEEN workshop report: Teaching and learning in interdisciplinary and empirical ethics. *Clinical Ethics*, 8, 70–74.

192 Andrew Papanikitas

James, H. S. & Rassekh, F. 2000. Smith, Friedman, and self-interest in ethical society. *Business Ethics Quarterly*, 10, 659–674.

Jani, A. & Papanikitas, A. 2018. "More than my job is worth" – Defensive medicine and the marketisation of healthcare. *In:* Feiler, T., Hordern, J. & Papanikitas, A. (eds.) *Marketisation, Ethics and Healthcare: Policy, Practice and Moral Formation.* Abingdon: Routledge.

Kerasidou, A. & Horn, R. 2018. Empathy in the healthcare system: Limits and scope of empathy in the public and private system. *In:* Feiler, T., Papanikitas, A. & Hordern, J. (eds.) *Marketisation, Ethics and Healthcare: Policy, Practice and Moral Formation.* Abingdon: Routledge.

McCullough, L. B. 2011. Was bioethics founded on historical and conceptual mistakes about medical paternalism? *Bioethics*, 25, 66–74.

Misselbrook, D. 2018. The virtuous professional and the marketplace. *In:* Feiler, T., Papanikitas, A. & Hordern, J. (eds.) *Marketisation, Ethics and Healthcare: Policy, Practice and Moral Formation.* Abingdon: Routledge.

NHS. 2017a. *Ethical Framework for Decision-Making* [Online]. North West London Collaboration of Clinical Commissioning Groups. Available: www.westlondonccg.nhs.uk/media/14695/06.3.f)%20Appendix%205%20-%20Ethical-framework.pdf [Accessed 14/8/2017].

NHS. 2017b. *Thames Valley Priorities Committee: Ethical Framework* [Online]. Thames Valley Priorities Committee. Available: www.fundingrequests.cscsu.nhs.uk/wp-content/uploads/2015/08/Ethical-Framework-March-2016-final.pdf [Accessed 14/08/2017].

Oswald, M. & Cox, D. 2011. Making difficult choices: Ethical commissioning guidance to general practitioners. *In:* RCGP (ed.). London: Royal College of General Practitioners.

Papanikitas, A. 2017a. The inescapability of conscience in primary healthcare. *In:* Papanikitas, A. & Spicer, J. (eds.) *Handbook of Primary Care Ethics.* Abingdon: CRC Press.

Papanikitas, A. 2017b. Self-awareness and professionalism. *InnovAiT*, 10, 452–457.

Papanikitas, A., De Zulueta, P., Spicer, J., Knight, R., Toon, P. & Misselbrook, D. 2011. Ethics of the ordinary: A meeting run by the royal society of medicine with the royal college of general practitioners. *London Journal of Primary Care*, 4, 70–72.

Papanikitas, A. & Spicer, J. 2017. Teaching and learning ethics in primary healthcare. *In:* Papanikitas, A. & Spicer, J. (eds.) *Handbook of Primary Care Ethics.* Abingdon: CRC Press.

Parker, J. 2017. *Reflections on Medical Ethics Teaching in the Foundation Years* [Online]. Researchgate. Available: www.researchgate.net/publication/319086201_Reflections_on_Medical_Ethics_Teaching_in_the_Foundation_Years [Accessed 14/08/2017].

Petrova, M., Dale, J. & Fulford, B. K. 2006. Values-based practice in primary care: Easing the tensions between individual values, ethical principles and best evidence. *British Journal of General Practice*, 56, 703–709.

Roland, M. 2012. Incentives must be closely aligned to professional values. *British Medical Journal*, 345, e5982.

Sandel, M. 2012. Two tenets of market faith. *In: What Money can't Buy: The Moral Limits of Markets.* London: Penguin.

Skinner, A. 1986. Introduction. *In:* Skinner, A. (ed.) *The Wealth of Nations Books I-III.* London: Penguin Classics.

Smith, A. 1759. *Of the Principle of Self-Approbation and of Self-Disapprobation* [Online]. Available: www.econlib.org/library/Smith/smMS3.html [Accessed 15/8/2017].

Sokol, D. 2016. Teaching medical ethics: Useful or useless? *BMJ*, 355, i6415.

Sokol, D. K. 2010. What to tell junior doctors about ethics. *BMJ*, 340, c2489.

Stirrat, G. M., Johnston, C., Gillon, R., Boyd, K., Medical Education Working Group of Institute of Medical, E. & Associated, S. 2010. Medical ethics and law for doctors of tomorrow: The 1998 consensus statement updated. *Journal of Medical Ethics*, 36, 55–60.

Toon, P. 1994. General practice as a business and patients as consumers. *In:* Perreira-Gray, D. (ed.) *What is Good General Practice?* London: Royal College of General Practitioners.

Toon, P. D. 2009. Towards an understanding of the flourishing practitioner. *Postgraduate Medical Journal*, 85, 399–403.

Toulmin, S. 1982. How medicine saved the life of ethics. *Perspectives in Biology and Medicine*, 25, 736–750.

Toynbee, M., Al-Diwani, A. A., Clacey, J. & Broome, M. R. 2016. Should junior doctors strike? *Journal of Medical Ethics*, 42, 167–170.

Wainwright, S. P., Williams, C., Michael, M., Farsides, B. & Cribb, A. 2006. Ethical boundary-work in the embryonic stem cell laboratory. *Sociology of Health and Illness*, 28, 732–748.

Walsh, A. 2018. Commercialisation and the corrosion of the ideals of medical professionals. *In:* Feiler, T., Hordern, J. & Papanikitas, A. (eds.) *Marketisation, Ethics and Healthcare: Policy, Practice and Moral Formation*. Abingdon: Routledge.

Wilson, D. 2014a. Criticising club regulation and "the birth of bioethics"? *In: The Making of British Bioethics*. Manchester: Manchester University Press.

Wilson, D. 2014b. "Who's for bioethics?" Ian Kennedy, oversight and accountability in the 1980s. *In: The Making of British Bioethics*. Manchester: Manchester University Press.

WT. 2017. *Seed Awards in Humanities and Social Science* [Online]. London: Wellcome Trust. Available: https://wellcome.ac.uk/funding/seed-awards-humanities-and-social-science [Accessed 14/8/2017].

What next? Editors' epilogue

In three parts, the chapters collated in this volume have covered three formal levels to consider when we talk about marketisation – systemic, policy and professionals. Each one of them has brought together similar, but also contrary and even opposed, understandings of what marketisation means and how we should work with the present situation. The following final thoughts from the editors indicate questions and ideas for further research.

Therese Feiler

For Therese Feiler, having engaged closely with Part I of this volume, one further route of enquiry concerns the evolving relationship between theology and different materialist schools of thought, in particular economics, Marxist theory and even a new 'speculative realism'. Recent movements in economics, for example the Cambridge Social Ontology Group, investigate social structures and 'existents' such as care, authority or profit as more ontologically fine-grained than we might be used to. This could well be made fruitful for the debate about the nature and institutional forms of healthcare from a systematic-theological and a religious-philosophical perspective. The connections between Marxism and theology remain equally illuminating, not least due to a shared radical scepticism. Of course, this connection is not new. The Jewish philosopher and lifelong 'left-wing oddball' Walter Benjamin, for example, said his 'thinking related to theology like the blotting paper relates to ink. It is saturated in it. Were one to go by the blotting paper, however, nothing of what is written would remain'. For all the rejections of Marxism, its influence remains subcutaneous but pervasive in movements such as 'Blue Labour' in English politics, or Pope Francis' proximity to liberation theology, indeed the living nineteenth-century roots of the welfare state as such. In this regard, somewhat free-floating political-philosophical and political-theological debates need to be critically interrogated more frequently with a view to their implications for healthcare and medicine.

Second, the present collection of essays has demonstrated different ways in which the stark contrast between, on the one hand, a total material(ist) market in medicine based on supply and demand, and on the other hand a purely gift-based, humanistic, indifferent care can be *mediated*. Petratos re-locates the question of justice to the outside of economics; instead of mediating between the two, he seeks to confine economics to the role of a limited tool. For Epstein, the humanist project is an open, frontal challenge and possibility, though he seems more open to effective and caring forms of 'false consciousness' than e.g. Marx would be. And whilst Hordern suggests that moral convictions and relationships should be made visible or fortified as a covenant, such a kind of first order representation or mediation can be compared to mediating organisations and structures such as those envisaged by Frith in Part I of the book. The nature, forms or failures of mediation thus require further consideration.

Finally, the nature of interdisciplinarity accompanies many multi-disciplinary projects, particularly when dealing with large-scale concepts such as marketisation. Over the decades, healthcare has seen a pluralisation of discourses very much in the postmodern sense, not only as a result of a pluralisation of medical specialties and organisational differentiation. One way to handle this might be to find a common language to debate marketisation. However, this contravenes the idea of multi-disciplinarity, perhaps creates a new managerial 'blob' and hence is intellectually unattractive. Differences between views, at least at this level of reflection, are not mere difference of opinion or taste, but a difference of ideas as theological, philosophical controversies throughout history. The terms and 'positions from which we speak' academically require – or at least imply – a (self-)positioning of disciplines vis-à-vis the object of research as such. A greater historical (self-)awareness, and a certain amount of what one might call scientific-academic self-sociology is therefore a future demand on collaborations between medicine, healthcare and academia.

Joshua Hordern

For Joshua Hordern, responsible especially for editing Part III of the volume but closely engaged also in Part II, a central thread of the volume which requires further research concerns the complexities of moral psychology at work in processes of marketisation. By 'moral psychology' here is meant reasons for belief and behaviour, and especially those which lie at the level of the affections – the loves which shape human reasoning and flourishing and which are commonly glossed as 'values'.

Systems and structures matter to moral psychology. They define what is normal and thinkable – they order that which should be valued. But what is normalised is not necessarily that which should be accepted. Therefore, systems and structures become that over against which resistance may be necessary at a moral-psychological level. It is all too easy to think that the organisational features of healthcare which present the greatest difficulties for the moral psychology of healthcare professionals and patients are those associated with what is assumed to be the inevitably pernicious effects of healthcare's marketisation healthcare.

However, what the different parts of the book may be taken to suggest is that what matters is how the underlying structures of healthcare, which take form in institutions, may or may not accommodate praiseworthy attitudes and behaviours.

And so neither does it seem true that marketisation is necessarily pernicious for healthcare, nor is it the case that everything stands and falls on the level of individual moral psychology. Organisational ethos and the culture in which organisations grow matter greatly for what groups of people come to love.

In all of this, there is something particularly compelling in the decentralising power of marketisation as narrated by Petratos, which distributes both the authority to determine what should count as valuable and the opportunity to do good works to enable that value to be experienced. Nonetheless, it is a matter of the first importance to cultivate a sober, realistic awareness about the dual tendencies towards self-deception and exploitation which characterise human life. We may be the more deceived about individuals' capacity to stand firm and make good choices to secure that which they value. For individuals and communities have to negotiate with those who would, for the sake of values of their own, perhaps reducible to mere financial value, exploit them with an eye to their main chance rather than their neighbour's good.

Nonetheless, the response to this is hardly to extirpate marketisation processes from healthcare. This would seem an incursion on the kind of human freedom which democracies ought to protect, which is unwarranted by the actual problems at stake. Rather it should be the case that the institutional forms of healthcare discipline and regulate practices which not only *assure* the keeping of contracts, but which also *encourage* the submission of such contractual relations, premised on financial exchange, to the higher order of a covenantal human relationship.

It is, therefore, the moral-psychological ordering of law, contract and regulation to the purposes of love, compassion and covenant which is at stake in how the marketisation of healthcare functions. This is necessary at an organisational and regulatory level, at the level of specific policy innovation and at the level of personal professional identity. How are the responsibility and self-management which characterises humanity at its best to walk hand in hand with the compassion which characterises humanity at its best? This is the problem which lies at the moral-psychological heart of marketisation in healthcare and to which many of the chapters in this volume give intriguing answers.

The complexities of evaluating what matters in human life can be supported, but are never exhausted by, processes of marketisation. The distribution of authority which markets enable towards the consumer and away from the central state can become a kind of end in itself as if this were true freedom. But the freedom which a certain kind of 'autonomy' envisages is hardly the social freedom, protected by law, to love and be loved which lies at the heart of humanity's vocation.

Andrew Papanikitas

For Andrew Papanikitas, working on this volume has been coloured by his experience as both a medical doctor and someone who teaches medical ethics to doctors and medical students.

This volume clarifies the idea that the market is a human tool rather than a force of nature – an artificial means of distributing resources. This much is clear in the chapters by Petratos and Epstein, though they argue for different ideologies and conclusions. The market is also a tool by which we understand the materiality of healthcare and indeed of morality applied to healthcare. Various chapters in this volume highlight how healthcare is reduced to economic units and the moral hazards that this simplification entails.

Such a reduction to economic units is difficult for two reasons. First, it strips away personhood from the persons and human narratives which are transvalued: people, illness, treatment and care are represented in economic terms (including as monetary amounts). It seems plausible that this stripping of personhood becomes less noticeable the further removed one is from the front line of healthcare delivery. Second, transvaluations are potentially incomplete and give the illusion of evidence-based scientific truth rather than units of worth that are heavily influenced by values and preferences.

The transvaluation of patients, illness and care is a reminder that, unless we foster both moral awareness and the will to engage with moral challenges, many, if not all, difficult decisions in healthcare will be resolved on economic grounds alone. The perennial fear with marketised healthcare is that people will be treated purely as means, and that money will become the sole end. The notion that a market in healthcare cannot be a completely rational market has implications for both healthcare purchaser and healthcare provider. Bilateral irrationality is here illustrated by defensive medicine. Both clinician and patient suffer. The patient suffers from healthcare that is 'mal-adapted' to protect healthcare from risk at the cost of good practice. The clinician suffers because both personal and institutional fear limits their potential to flourish in their art. The market is distorted by providers who shy away from those who need healthcare most, and who offer health tests and treatments that patients do not need.

Thinking about the many stakeholders in healthcare (framed as a market) rehearses the idea that morality is not just about those who are 'done to', but those who are called upon to 'do'. In this volume, a recurring theme has been the respect for persons, which ought to be a respect for *all* persons – and not only the purchaser, or the end-user of healthcare. The message that ethics itself is a potential instrument of oppression by employers, or even governments, stands alongside the message that reflexive, reasoned morality is an antidote to the corrupting influence of wealth, described almost as an illness that Walsh in this volume calls 'lucrepathy'. If reasoning and reflection have a role to play in safeguarding the souls of healthcare professionals and the lives and health of patients, then care needs to be taken to ensure this activity is protected. The economic value and the material impacts of healthcare ethics activities are critically in need of further study. Some work has been done on who buys bioethics research, but this needs further research. Work on the place and value of other activities such as consultancy, teaching and practical ethics support in a healthcare market seems virtually non-existent.

Codes, convenants, compassion, conscience, conversation and more solutions are offered in the preceding chapters. All are important. And if this collection illustrates anything, it is that one easy process will not provide the answer to the question of how to live with a healthcare marketplace. All, however, are activities that should have material effects on the world. As such they are very much a part of the market that they seek to civilise. If we are sincere in that respect for persons which is the ostensible basis for democratic society and healthcare ethics, then money should be a means, and people should be ends in themselves. And if we understand how the things that should never be bought and sold connect with the material world, there is a chance they remain visible – even to those who now see the price of everything and the value of nothing.

Index

Tables are indicated by page numbers in **bold** type; figures are indicated by page numbers in *italic* type.

202   *Index*

organisational ethics 49–64, 196;
  background 49–51; critical 59–61;
  developing 57–59; ethical aspects of
  51–53; growth of 53–54; programmes
  55–57; relationships 54–55
organ transplantation 43–44, 138
orientations 185
OS (organization studies) 60
outsourcing 26, 44

Pabst, A. 152
Palestine 72
Papanikitas, A. 6, 8, 127, 177, 196–198
Pareto, V. 17, 28
Pareto optimal 17
pastoral theology 112–113, 121, 128
paternalism 71, 88, 101, 121, 183
pathology 149
patient-as-consumer 113
patient-centredness 68, 76, 149–151,
  176, 180
Patient-Physician Covenant 120–121,
  148–153
patient/population-outcomes 107
patients 33–35, 36, 43, 54, 71, 75, 101,
  120, 171
Paul, the apostle 78
payers 102–103
Payment by Results (PbR) 68, 71
payments 85–86, 107, 127, 134, **176**
Pellegrino, E. 157–158, 164, 169
Pennsylvania study 99
personal assistant model 90–91
personalisation 88–89
perspectives 168–171
Petratos, P. 3–4, 51, 53, 73, 114, 116, 194,
  196, 197
PFI (Public Finance Initiatives) 51
Pharma 159
philanthropy 28–29, 143
philosophical question 40, 45n12
phronesis 156–157, 160
physicians 33–36, 99–100, 119–121
Pinsent, A. 153
Plasma Resources UK 50
Plato 137
pleasure of health 13
plenitude 70, 72, 75–76, 114
pluralisation 2
pluralist health system 21
policies: academic studies 182; in Australia
  134; defining 3; in England 49–51;
  ethics 181–184; social 69; spending
  87–88; trust 127

polis 7, 147, 155–156, 158–159
politics 2, 5, 8, 28, 71–74, 79–80, 80n4,
  111–113, 135
Pol Pot 155
pooling 22–24
Powell, M. 50
power 37–39, 51, 59, 150
preference utilitarianism 13–14, 21, 24
prejudices 168
price-dignity dictum 139–140
pricing 17–18, 20, 43, 139, 145n6
Primary Care Trusts 50
Priorities Support Unit 180
privacy 42
private healthcare systems 22, 163, 165–168
private insurance model 22
private sector 49
privatisation 27, 34, 44, 50
production 14, 16–18, 138
productivity 52
professionalism 52, 55, 116; *see also* virtue
professional legal representative 43
profit motive 120, 134–135, 137–138,
  140–144
profits: abnormal 4; calculating 16;
  corruption and 35; determining 67; as
  ends in themselves 140; ethics and 36;
  generating 104, 114, 120; legitimate
  152; and moral values 7, 144–145;
  normal 14
programmes, organisational ethics
  55–57, 60
property 14, 50, 167
Proverbs 70
providers 49
provision 21–22, 22–24
psychology 37–38, 45n9, 195–196
public-economics model 53
Public Finance Initiatives (PFI) 51
public healthcare systems 163, 165–168
purchasing 22–24
Putting People First (DoH) 88

quality 76, 84
Quality-Adjusted Life-Years (QALYs) 42,
  74–76
Quality Outcome Framework (QOF)
  150, 160

Rassekh, F. 176
rationality 38, 45n7, 185
rationing 42–43
Rawls, J. 153, 159–160; *A Theory of
  Justice* 136

For Product Safety Concerns and Information please contact our
EU representative GPSR@taylorandfrancis.com Taylor & Francis
Verlag GmbH, Kaufingerstraße 24, 80331 München, Germany